Statistics in Psychiatry

Arnold Applications of Statistics Series

Series Editor: **BRIAN EVERITT**
Department of Biostatistics and Computing, Institute of Psychiatry, London, UK

This series offers titles which cover the statistical methodology most relevant to particular subject matters. Readers will be assumed to have a basic grasp of the topics covered in most general introductory statistics courses and texts, thus enabling the authors of the books in the series to concentrate on those techniques of most importance in the discipline under discussion. Although not introductory, most publications in the series are applied rather than highly technical, and all contain many detailed examples.

Other titles in the series:

Statistics in Education Ian Plewis

Statistics in Civil Engineering Andrew Metcalfe

Statistics in Human Genetics Pak Sham

Statistics in Finance Edited by David Hand & Saul Jacka

Statistics in Sport Edited by Jay Bennett

Statistics in Society Edited by Daniel Dorling & Stephen Simpson

Statistics in Psychiatry

Graham Dunn
Biostatistics Group, University of Manchester

A member of the Hodder Headline Group
LONDON
Copublished in the United States of America by
Oxford University Press Inc., New York

First published in Great Britain in 2000 by Arnold,
a member of the Hodder Headline Group,
338 Euston Road, London NW1 3BH

http://www.arnoldpublishers.com

Copublished in the United States of America by
Oxford University Press Inc.,
198 Madison Avenue, New York, NY10016

British Library Cataloguing in Publication Data
A catalogue record for this book is available from the British Library

Library of Congress Cataloging-in-Publication Data
A catalog record for this book is available from the Library of Congress

ISBN 0 340 67668 X

1 2 3 4 5 6 7 8 9 10

Commissioning Editor: Nicki Dennis
Production Editor: Rada Radojicic
Production Controller: Iain McWilliams
Cover Design: M2

Typeset in 10/11 Times by Academic & Technical Typesetting, Bristol
Printed and bound in Great Britain by J W Arrowsmith Ltd, Bristol

What do you think about this book? Or any other Arnold title?
Please send your comments to feedback.arnold@hodder.co.uk

Contents

Preface

In writing this book my aim has been to create an intermediate text suitable for practising research workers in psychiatry and related disciplines. It is intended for clinical, behavioural or social scientists, as well as applied statisticians with limited experience in the mental health field. The style is problem-based rather than technique-led. Having said that, however, the choice of research problems is made with a view to the techniques used to solve them. The title *Statistics in Psychiatry* should perhaps be interpreted as *Statistics in Psychiatric Epidemiology*, thus better reflecting both the book's content and the interests and experience of its author. Readers looking for a technical discussion of genetic linkage, for example, or a statistical introduction to brain imaging, will be disappointed. Although I had originally intended to include a fairly lengthy discussion of clinical trial methodology, this too was eventually jettisoned in favour of more material on observational studies. I make no apology for this – a book of this kind cannot be expected to cover everything of relevance to research into mental illness and the selection of topics is inevitably a personal one. I have tried to select topics for chapters that will reveal the distinctive 'flavour' of the subject. And the flavour is completely dominated by the problems of measurement error. A statistician working in the mental health field will inevitably use many of the techniques common to medical statistics in general. But it would have been a bit pointless (for the author at least!) writing a standard medical statistics text which differs from its competitors not in terms of the topics covered but merely in the selection of examples to illustrate the use of the techniques. At the very least, the present text will be something different. I hope that my selection of topics will be seen by its readers as one of the book's strengths rather than its weakness.

The ideas for much of the material in this book have arisen through close collaboration with clinical colleagues. A glance at the illustrative examples in several of the chapters will reveal that I am particularly indebted to Glyn Lewis (University of Wales), Michele Tansella (University of Verona) and José Luis Vázquez-Barquero (University of Cantabria). I thank them both for letting me use their data so extensively and also for providing me with such stimulating problems in the first place.

I would particularly like to acknowledge the influence over many years of my statistical colleagues Brian Everitt (Institute of Psychiatry) and Andrew Pickles (University of Manchester). Before Andrew and I left the Institute of Psychiatry and moved north to Manchester, the three of us ran regular short courses on modelling covariance matrices and latent variables in EQS. Over the last few years Andrew and I have also collaborated on multiphase sampling problems. They have both read and commented on large parts of the current text, although I accept full responsibility for the choice of material and any errors that might have appeared despite their efforts.

I would also like to thank David Hand (Open University) and Pak Sham (Institute of Psychiatry) for agreeing to let me use a lot of the material from our review on statistics and the nature of depression (Dunn, Sham and Hand, 1993) in the introductory chapter of the present work.

Several people have read various drafts of some of the chapters and I would like to thank them for their input. In particular, I would like to thank Melanie Abbas (Institute of Psychiatry) who read preliminary drafts of some of the earlier chapters. Although she was quite complimentary about them it was her comments (together with some of Brian Everitt's) that prompted me to discard these early efforts and start again. I then realised that it would be point-less to try to be comprehensive and that what I should be doing was attempting to write something different. But, of course, I fully accept responsibility for the choice of topics in the final version! Partly as a result of this change of direction the book has taken me much longer to write than I had originally planned and I would like to thank Brian Everitt (the editor of the series) and Nicki Dennis (from Arnold, the publishers) for their patience.

Finally, I would like to thank my wife Jane for putting up with so many work-ing weekends in which I struggled to think what to write next.

Graham Dunn
April 1999

'Such a disease, which disorders the senses, perverts the reason and breaks up the passions in wild confusion – which assails man in his essential nature – brings down so much misery on the head of its victims, and is productive of so much social evil – deserves investigation on its own merits, by statistical as well as by other methods.... We may discover the causes of insanity, the laws which regulate its course, the circumstances by which it is influenced, and either avert its visitations, or mitigate their severity; perhaps in a later age, save mankind from its inflictions, or if this cannot be, at any rate ensure the sufferers early treatment.' (Sir William Farr, 1841)

1

Introduction

1.1 Statistics and psychiatry

I start by following Kramer (1989) in quoting the report of the Milbank Memorial Fund Commission on 'Higher Education in Public Health' (Milbank Memorial Fund Commission, 1972, p. 62):

Biostatistics uses statistical methodology to investigate problems in public health and medical care. In addition to collecting, analyzing, and retrieving data, designing experiments, and developing appropriate comparisons among population groups, biostatistics applies the techniques of inference and probability to the examination of biologic data. While interacting most continuously and closely with epidemiology, biostatistic interests extend into the congruent areas of vital statistics and demography, computer programming, computer systems and analysis, and program planning evaluation. Through the continuing collaboration of epidemiologists and biostatisticians, the science and skill of designing experiments, analytic surveys, and data analysis have progressed to an advanced level. The actual work of these two types of specialists mesh so closely at times that it may be difficult for the outsider to distinguish between them. Through a fruitful working relationship, each in fact has come to learn a great deal about the other's methods and activities. Both as an arm of epidemiology and as a separate science, biostatistics serves as the major method of quantifying and analyzing health information specifically for application within public health.

Now, this is a pretty good description of the activities of a medical statistician – but how well does it describe the activities, for example, of a biostatistician in London's Institute of Psychiatry or a similar institution in continental Europe or the USA? Not very well – it is incomplete. Psychiatry is more than a branch of medicine and psychiatric epidemiology is an extremely rich mix of traditional chronic disease epidemiology, social science and psychology, in which multivariate statistical methods play a central and prominent role. Statisticians in this area typically use a much wider variety of multivariate statistical methods than do medical statisticians elsewhere. Scientific psychiatry has always taken the problems of measurement much more seriously than appears to be the case in other clinical specialties. This is partly due to the fact that the measurement problems in psychiatry are obviously rather complex, but partly also because the other clinical fields appear to have been a bit backward by comparison. It is also an academic discipline where, at its best, there is fruitful interplay between the ideas typical of the 'medical model' of disease and those coming from the psychometric traditions of, say, educationalists and personality theorists.

> Mental diseases have both psychological, sociological and biological aspects and their study requires a combination of the approaches of the psychologist, the sociologist and the biologist, using the last word rather than physician since the latter must be all three. In *each* of these aspects statistical reasoning plays an essential part, whether it be in the future planning of hospitals, the classification of the various forms of such illnesses, the study of causation or the evaluation of methods of treatment. (Moran, 1969 – my italics).

> Possibly because it frightens us all to some extent, psychiatric medicine has never been a popular subject for research and it is only of fairly recent years that there has been a sufficient volume of medical work for the statistical world as a whole to get its teeth into. Unfortunately, many of the statistical problems that arise (or at any rate those that the psychiatrists have chosen to study) are exceedingly difficult ones, and psychiatrists have often taken over from psychology an armoury of powerful but imperfectly understood techniques; some of the resulting work has led more to controversy than clarification. (Healy, 1969).

Healy's comment is probably still true 30 years on. Moran (1969), for example, described some of the controversies concerning the classification of depression. They can also be found in Dunn, Sham and Hand (1993) and in later sections of the present chapter. For further discussion of the role of statistics in psychiatry, I refer the reader to articles by Everitt (1987) and Everitt and Landau (1998) and to a special issue of *Statistical Methods in Medical Research* (October 1998).

In what follows, the reader should not be expecting to see descriptions of standard techniques from medical statistics applied to data on mental illness. This would be a bit pointless. Instead of this I have chosen to select a variety of statistical approaches which can be very powerful tools for the psychiatric epidemiologist and which emphasise the distinct characteristics of the discipline. The aetiology of mental illness inevitably involves complex and inadequately understood interactions between social stressors and genetically and socially determined vulnerabilities – the whole area being overlaid by a thick carpet of measurement and misclassification errors. Social, educational and behavioural statisticians will probably feel more at home here than medical statisticians and traditionally trained epidemiologists but it is to be hoped that the latter will find the unfamiliar material more of an exciting challenge than something to be wary of.

1.2   Measurement

The role and importance of measurement in scientific psychiatry is too obvious to need labouring here. Multidimensional measurement is needed for the purpose of a full characterisation of a particular form of mental illness or handicap, for diagnosis and classification, for the evaluation of treatment or care, and so on. The variety of characteristics that can be measured, and frequently are measured, is vast. There is also a wide variety of methods available to assess each of these characteristics. They could be based on patients' self-reports, behavioural observations, the reports of key informants such as close relatives or care staff, or the judgement of clinicians and other professionals involved in the management of the patients. Many of these methods involve the use of rating scales, with the data being collected through the use of questionnaires and structured interviews.

Rather than attempting to draw up a comprehensive list of measuring instruments, I will simply illustrate the point by reference to the list of symptom and functioning measures used in a recent randomised controlled trial to evaluate cognitive–behavioural therapy for psychosis (Kuipers *et al.*, 1997):

> We used the Present State Examination (PSE-10, World Health Organisation, 1992) to establish psychotic symptomatology, using the associated CATEGO-V programme to derive diagnostic categories according to DSM-III-R (American Psychiatric Association, 1987) at baseline. The Brief Psychiatric Rating Scale (19-item, 0–6 scale) (BPRS; Overall and Gorham, 1962) was administered to assess overall mental state (baseline and three-monthly). . . . We used Personal Questionnaires every three months to monitor changes in key symptoms identified by the PSE, as this methodology has proved to be both reliable and sensitive (Brett-Jones *et al.*, 1987). For delusions we measured conviction, preoccupation and distress; for hallucinations we measured frequency, intensity and distress. We also assessed hallucinations (Hustig and Hafner, 1990) three-monthly, and used the Maudsley Assessment of Delusions Schedule (MADS; Buchanan *et al.*, 1993) (baseline and nine months).
>
> Insight (Amador *et al.*, 1993) was measured at baseline and at nine months. The Beck Depression Inventory (BDI; Beck *et al.*, 1961) (three-monthly), the Beck Anxiety Inventory (BAI; Beck *et al.*, 1988), Beck Hopelessness Scale (BHS; Beck *et al.*, 1974) (baseline and nine months), and the Social Functioning Scale (Birchwood *et al.*, 1990) (baseline and nine months) were completed.

As well as these symptom and function measures, Kuipers *et al.* also assessed various cognitive deficits in their patients, together with their self-esteem, dysfunctional attitudes and satisfaction with therapy. They could have included the assessment of the patients' needs, quality of life, social disability, caregiver burden and much more (see, for example, Thornicroft and Tansella, 1996).

Several of the chapters of the present book concentrate on statistical methods to evaluate the properties (mainly in terms of reliability and validity) of various psychiatric rating scales, case-finding instruments and diagnostic interviews. In fact, the whole of the book is dominated by the problems of evaluating and allowing for measurement errors of various kinds. There are many aspects of instrument development that are not covered, however. Some of them are briefly introduced in the present chapter, mainly to set the scene for the rest of the book. Again, rather than trying to be comprehensive, we will concentrate on measures of symptom severity and, in particular, the measurement of depression and anxiety. Much of the material on depression is based on the review by Dunn, Sham and Hand (1993).

1.2.1   Historical foundations

The discipline of psychology was one of the first to make thorough use of the statistical methods developed at the beginning of the present century. The first edition of William Brown's book *The Essentials of Mental Measurement* (Brown, 1911) appeared in the same year as G. Udny Yule's *An Introduction to the Theory of Statistics* (Yule, 1911). The purpose of Brown's book was to make the then new biometrical methods of Galton, Pearson and Yule more generally known among psychologists. The other major proponent of the use of correlational methods at that time was Charles Spearman. Spearman is well known amongst statisticians and psychologists as the originator of factor analysis (see Spearman, 1904). The pioneering studies of Spearman and Brown (see, for example, Spearman, 1910; Brown, 1910) together with slightly later ones in the United States by Truman Kelley (Kelley, 1923) formed the foundations of what is now known as 'classical test theory' (see Chapter 2).

Rather surprisingly, however, these developments had very little impact on the outlook of clinicians working in the superficially related field of psychiatry. Why this is so is not at all clear. Brown himself was clinically trained and at one time held an appointment as Resident Medical Officer at the Maudsley Hospital and directed research in clinical psychology at the Bethlem Hospital (Burt, 1952). Bernard Hart, an early collaborator with Spearman (Hart and Spearman, 1912), was also a psychiatrist.

The first publication on correlation in psychiatry seems to have been a paper on perseveration by the psychologist L.L. Wynn Jones (Wynn Jones, 1928) in the *Journal of Mental Science* (the forerunner of the *British Journal of Psychiatry*). This paper includes a technical footnote on the calculations of Pearson's product–moment correlation coefficient. The same volume of this journal also contains Edwin Mapother's review of Spearman's *The Abilities of Man* (Mapother, 1928; Spearman, 1927). Mapother was clearly quite impressed by Spearman's work: 'It seems quite likely that this book might have upon normal and morbid psychology the sort of influence that the "Origin of Species" has in biology.' He goes on to state that 'It is especially desirable that workers trained in the analysis of mental functions upon the lines indicated by Prof. Spearman should co-operate with clinicians in defining the problems of both normal psychology and psychiatry and in attempts at their solution.' And, finally, he says the book's 'trend is above all to ensure the substitution of measurement for uncontrolled assertion – a consummation that is overdue in psychiatry'.

In 1929 Spearman delivered the Tenth Maudsley Lecture: 'The Psychiatric Use of the Methods and Results of Experimental Psychology'. At the end of this lecture he proposed that clinicians and experimental psychologists should undertake joint research in which 'a carefully chosen group of patients be submitted to observation and measurement of every feasible kind' (Spearman, 1929). This work was started under the supervision of Spearman and the psychiatrist J.R. Lord and the first of a series of five papers on 'Studies in experimental psychiatry' was published by W. Stephenson in 1931 (see Stephenson, 1931, 1932a, 1932b; Simins, 1933; and Studman, 1935). This burst of activity, however, did not lead directly to work on the measurement of the severity of symptoms. Stephenson and his colleagues were primarily interested in the cognitive and conative characteristics of the patients. Later work concentrated on the measurement of temperament or personality (see, for example, Burt, 1940). The work is, however, indicative of a profound change of attitude in some areas of psychiatric research (see also Ellund and Doering, 1928). Psychiatrists, or at least the psychologists working with them, had started to attempt to use objective methods of measurement and to assess their value by statistical techniques.

The first attempt at construction of a questionnaire and corresponding rating scale for the measurement of depression appears to have been that of Jasper at the University of Iowa (Jasper, 1930). Although Jasper was attempting to measure a depressive temperament in normal healthy adults rather than the depth of depression in patients, his work can be regarded as the forerunner of more recent work on psychiatric rating scales. Jasper was clearly influenced by Spearman's common factor theory in his understanding of the concept of depression as being analogous to the cognitive characteristic, which Spearman called 'general intelligence'. He also used the statistical methods of Spearman, Brown and Kelley in order to assess the reliability and validity of the newly derived measure of depression–elation. This early work on the objective measurement of depression is typical of the use made of statistical ideas in evaluating the rating scale as it was being developed. These methods were to be used over and over again in the work on the measurement of the severity of depression that was to be published over 30 years later.

1.2.2 The development and evaluation of rating scales for depression

Modern rating scales for depression are basically of two types: self-assessment through the use of a questionnaire, and assessment by a clinician following a psychiatric interview. The Beck Depression Inventory (BDI) is the most commonly used example of the former (Beck *et al.*, 1961). The Hamilton Rating Scale (HRS) for depression is regarded as the standard scale of the latter type (Hamilton, 1960, 1967). There are, of course, many other rating scales and screening instruments for the detection and measurement of depressive symptoms now available, but here we will concentrate on the BDI and the HRS only. For a more general review the reader is directed to Mayer (1978) and Bech (1981).

The usual form of the HRS consists of 17 items covering symptoms of depression, with the severity of depression being calculated as the sum of the scores on these 17 items (Hamilton, 1967). Nine of the items are rated on a five-point ordinal scale and eight are rated on a three-point scale. The total score obtained through the use of the HRS is the sum of two independent ratings, one by the interviewer and the other by an observer, and can range from 0 to 100.

The BDI contains 21 items. Each item consists of a graded series of four or five alternative statements ranging from neutral (rated as 0) to a maximum level of severity (rated as 3) and the patient is asked to select the single statement within each item that corresponds most closely to his or her condition. As with the HRS, the total BDI score is obtained by adding the scores from the 21 items. The range of the total BDI score is for 0 to a maximum of 63. The characteristics of the HRS and BDI were, of course, originally studied using the methods of classical test theory.

1.2.3 Factor analysis and the internal structure of rating scales

Having developed a questionnaire or rating scale for depression it seems to be quite natural and justified to ask whether a single concept is being measured or whether there is more than one. Factor analysis is obviously an appropriate tool to use to explore this question. Here, as in the text by Bartholomew (1987), the term 'factor analysis' is taken to include measurement models for binary and categorical ratings (item response theory) as well as the classical model of Spearman and his successors. Many of the users of allied statistical techniques, such as principal components analysis and correspondence analysis, also view these as factor analytic methods and in fact these methods typically yield results that are very similar to those produced through the exploratory use of the corresponding factor model. Again, we will illustrate some of these developments from work on the internal structure of rating scales for depression.

Hamilton (1960, 1967) described principal components analyses of the Hamilton Rating Scale for depression. In separate analyses of correlation matrices for 152 men and 120 women, Hamilton (1967) investigated the first six principal components (out of a possible 17), these being the ones with eigenvalues greater than one. These six principal components were then subjected to an orthogonal rotation using the Varimax criterion. An attempt to replicate Hamilton's 1967 findings was reported by Mowbray (1972) who carried out a principal components analysis on correlation matrices from 134 male and 213 female depressed patients. Mowbray also attempted to simplify the interpretation of the results through the use of Varimax rotation of the largest principal components.

Both authors found a general 'factor', which could be labelled 'severity of depression'. From then on, however, the two sets of analyses diverge. Basically, the items of the rating scales are always positively correlated, but the exact pattern of the sizes of these correlations differs from one study to another. This can arise because of sampling fluctuations (exaggerated by the use of relatively small sample sizes) and also from the fact that different authors are sampling from different patient populations. Patient heterogeneity is also a significant problem. The outcome of these and other further analytic studies (see Bech, 1981) is very confusing. The results differ from one sample to another and are rather difficult to interpret. Similar comments also apply to factor analytic work on the Beck Depression Inventory (see Beck and Beamesderfer, 1974; Weckowicz *et al.*, 1978; and Bech, 1981). Some of the difficulties in the use of traditional factor analytic techniques in a dimensional description of psychiatric symptomatology are discussed in Maxwell (1972) and others are discussed in Boyle (1985) and Bech (1981). Much of the interesting recent work on the internal structure of rating scales has concentrated on the use of item response theory models (Rasch, 1960; Bartholomew, 1987, 1996) – see, for example, Bech (1981).

1.2.4   Diagnostic interview schedules and screening questionnaires

Modern surveys of adult psychiatric morbidity (and many other research studies) utilise essentially three types of case-finding or diagnostic instrument. The 'gold standard' is the structured diagnostic interview schedule that is administered by a fully trained and experienced clinician. Two of the best-known examples are the PSE (Present State Examination – see Wing *et al.*, 1974) and the SCAN (Schedules for Clinical Assessment in Neuropsychiatry – see Wing *et al.*, 1990). Wing (1996) describes the developmental history of these two instruments. A further example is Goldberg's CIS (Clinical Interview Schedule), which was designed for use in primary-care settings and community surveys (see Goldberg *et al.*, 1970). All of these are dependent on expert clinical judgement for their valid use. The major disadvantage of these 'gold standard' interview schedules is the cost of their use. This cost can be reduced in two ways. One approach is to develop two-phase sampling strategies in which everyone selected for the first-phase sample is asked to complete a simple and inexpensive screening questionnaire. The results of the first phase are then used to stratify the respondents, and sub-samples of these strata are then selected for a second-phase interview (see Chapter 5). The other approach to cost reduction is to develop interview schedules that can be administered by 'lay' interviewers (i.e. non-clinicians who have been specifically trained to carry out the case-finding interview). Examples of diagnostic interview schedules which have been designed for possible use by non-clinicians are the CIS-R (the Clinical Interview Schedule Revised – Lewis *et al.*, 1992), the DIS (Diagnostic Interview Schedule – Robins *et al.*, 1981) and the CIDI (Composite International Diagnostic Interview – Robins *et al.*, 1988).

Perhaps the best known of the screening questionnaires is the GHQ (General Health Questionnaire – Goldberg, 1972; Goldberg and Williams, 1988). Other example are the CES-D (Centre for Epidemiological Studies Depression Scale – Radloff, 1977) and the HADS (Hospital Anxiety and Depression Scale – Zigmond and Snaith, 1983). Occasionally a rating scale such as the BDI is also used as a screening instrument. Note that it is possible to use two or more screening instruments in the first phase of a two-phase survey and one also has the choice of using either a lay-administered interview at the second phase or the more expensive interview administered by a clinician. These and other complex multiphase assessment strategies have been advocated and described by Dohrenwend (1995).

Most of the above instruments will make an appearance in the rest of this book. It is not necessary for the reader to know their detailed contents or details of their administration. Those readers who might want further information, however, are referred to the historical review by Murphy (1995) and to selected chapters in Thornicroft and Tansella (1996).

Before we move on, however, let us emphasise that these instruments are simply a mechanism for obtaining essentially a profile of symptoms (either in terms of their presence or absence, or in terms of their severities). Moving from this profile of symptoms to some form of categorisation (diagnosis) or overall severity rating is an inference (or even an imposition) that may or may not be warranted. Quoting Wing (1996, p. 125):

> One unexpected problem was appreciated only after long use. There was a tendency to regard the computerised output from PSE9 only in terms of a single diagnosis rather than as a rich and varied psychometric profile. This was far from the authors' intention (Wing, 1983, 1994). A central principle was that the system could not 'make a diagnosis' in the straightforward clinical sense. The people who use it are responsible for interpreting the results according to their judgement of the adequacy of the interview, the quality of the data recorded and the choice of outputs categories. A 'final' category can be derived and interpreted as a diagnosis if the clinician so decides, but that decision is not made by the PSE or by the computer.
> Rose (1992) has made the point that diagnosis 'splits the world into two'; those who have and those who do not have a disorder. However, most problems have continuous distributions. The PSE was not originally designed as a diagnostic instrument but, in the course of its development as a comprehensive clinical tool, it came to provide a database capable (in addition to its psychometric properties) of expanding the more exacting algorithms presented in DSM-III.

The justification of 'splitting the world into two' is the subject of the following section.

1.3   Case-definition and diagnosis: categories or continua?

> Clinical diagnosis splits the world into two: with regard to each disease there are those who have it and those who do not. This dichotomy serves well enough in clinical practice, both because treatment decisions are dichotomous and selective referral brings to the doctor only the more severe examples of a condition. . . . In population studies the situation is not like this, and rating scales for mental illness show continuous, uni-modal distributions. 'It follows that to ask what fraction of a population is psychiatrically disturbed is a meaningless question' (Goldberg, 1972: 3). This is, nevertheless, exactly what most surveys have attempted to do, because the investigators were determined to force on to the population those descriptive labels with which they are clinically familiar. (Rose, 1989, pp. 78–79).

Rose goes on to compare this situation with essential hypertension and alcohol abuse, quoting Pickering:

> essential hypertension is a type of disease not hitherto recognised in medicine in which the defect is quantitative not qualitative. It is difficult for doctors to understand because it is a departure from the ordinary process of binary thought to which they are brought up. Medicine in its present state can count up to two but not beyond. (Pickering, 1968, p. 4).

According to Rose, and to many psychologists such as Eysenck (1970), it makes much more sense to think of continua rather than discrete classes. The question should be 'How much has he got?' rather than 'Has he got it?' (Rose, 1989, p. 79). This approach, of course, is much more in line with the psychometric traditions of Brown and Spearman and their many successors than it is with the more traditional medical model referred to by Pickering. In the previous section we quoted Wing stating that the PSE was designed to provide a rich and varied psychometric profile – not just a single psychiatric diagnosis. Both Wing and Rose (1989), quite justifiably, regard the extraction of a single diagnosis from interview schedules such as the PSE as a waste of information. 'Case definition may be necessary for operational decisions (as in screening), but it is too inefficient to earn priority in research: a distribution should always be analysed first by statistics which describe its central tendency and its dispersion' (Rose, 1989, p. 79).

Now, if we accept that the distinction between 'cases' and 'non-cases' is an arbitrary and operational one, we are likely to recognise that when it comes to attempts at classifying, say, depressives or schizophrenics into sub-types on the basis of their symptom profiles the outcome is likely to be just as arbitrary (and perhaps more so) and, again, a rather inefficient use of data. It is not surprising that these attempts have been both controversial and not very fruitful (see the following two sections for further details). When it comes to simultaneously classifying survey participants into several arbitrary clinical categories – 'depressed' vs. 'non-depressed', 'anxious' vs. 'not anxious', 'alcoholic' vs. 'non-alcoholic' (or even 'hypertensive' vs. 'non-hypertensive') – in so-called co-morbidity studies (see, for example, Kessler, 1994), then the problems of interpretation are likely to be rather difficult, to say the least. Here the traditional medical model becomes even more difficult to sustain.

Another area where the idea of splitting the world into two appears to lack any firm foundation is in the analysis and interpretation of the results of clinical trials and other intervention studies. Classifying the treated patients as 'cured' or 'not-cured' very rarely has any empirical or theoretical justification. Many if not most randomised controlled trials (RCTs) evaluate treatments using quantitative outcome measures (see, for example, the cognitive therapy trial of Kuipers *et al.*, 1997, quoted in Section 1.2). Patients may or may not benefit from the treatment or care they receive in a clinical trial but they very rarely make a full recovery. It is usually a case of degree and of whether the average improvement is better in one arm of the trial than in another. Fortunately most of these trials are actually analysed using statistical methodologies appropriate for quantitative outcome data. The problem arises in subsequent systematic reviews and associated meta-analyses when the reviewers (usually trained by general physicians using an invalid and inappropriate medical model for behavioural and other psychiatric problems) then insist on dichotomising outcomes. They then often have the cheek to complain that the original trials have been analysed in the incorrect way. This is nonsense! Binary outcomes should be imposed on quantitative data only with extreme care. Problems of 'case' definition are just as difficult, and the valid solution of these is perhaps even more important for the interpretation of trials than it is for the interpretation of epidemiological survey data.

1.3.1   Two types of depression?

Many different classification schemes have been proposed for depressive illness. Writing in 1976, Kendell remarked that:

> almost every classificatory format that is logically possible has been advocated by someone within the last twenty years. . . . There are classifications of depression embracing one, two, three, four, five, seven, eight or nine categories. Indeed Rumke (1960) recognised thirteen. Some are tiered, others are not. There are also dimensional classifications, with varying number of dimensions. (Kendell, 1976).

Particularly prominent are proposals for two sub-types. These go under various names: 'psychotic' versus 'neurotic', 'exogenous' versus 'endogenous', 'reactive' versus 'endogenous', and so on. The sort of features thought to distinguish endogenous (psychotic) depression from the exogenous (reactive, neurotic) form are the following. The former tends to be severe, unvarying, and accompanied by guilt, severe insomnia and weight loss. The latter consists of milder symptoms, varying from day to day, and accompanied by anxiety and self-pity. From these two descriptions it will be clear why some authors regard the two 'types' as being opposite poles in a continuum of severity. Perhaps we should also point out here that not all authors have used these names in the same way. Kendell (1976), in his excellent review of the classification of depression suggests that the confusion is so great that it might be best to abandon the above terms and begin anew. Readers are also referred to Kendell (1968). Manic-depressive illness has also been divided into two categories: 'bipolar', indicating alternating mania and depression, and 'unipolar', indicating recurrent depression or recurrent mania.

The controversies over the nature of depression can be summarised as follows:

> they are chiefly concerned with whether depression is unitary or binary, that is, a single syndrome or two syndromes (endogenous and reactive), and whether the syndrome or syndromes is/are categorical or dimensional, that is, whether they are discrete entities (categorical) or whether they are normally distributed and occur in varying combination with each other or with other syndromes (dimensional). (Becker, 1974, p. 38).

Note that two questions are being addressed here. One concerns the existence of clusters of individuals in the measurement space (categorical), and the other concerns the existence of distinct clusters of variables (dimensional). In each case the question is whether one or two clusters exist. (If, in fact, more than two clusters exist – if there are more than two types of depression – then this will complicate the issue considerably!) Much of the controversy in the area can be traced to a confusion between these two distinct questions. A factor analysis of symptoms, for example, tells us about the dimensionality of the symptom 'space', but it says nothing about the clustering of patients. We will not review the results of these studies here (see Dunn, Sham and Hand, 1993), but simply note that the controversies were never resolved.

It is clear that while the use of multivariate methods has not led to a solution of the controversy it may have led to a clearer understanding of the problem (Paykel, 1981). The work on the classification of patients with depression illustrates many of the faults characteristic of large areas of psychiatric research. The aims of the research tend to be rather poorly defined. It only makes sense to commit a lot of resources into searching for two types of depression if depression itself can be demonstrated to be distinct from other psychiatric disorders such as anxiety and schizophrenia (Kendell, 1976). If one chooses to use sophisticated multivariate statistical methods to solve a problem then it is vital that these methods should be used appropriately and correctly. Even the lack of understanding of the causes and implications of the relatively simple concept of bimodality has caused much confusion – despite frequent warnings (see, for example, Murphy (1964), Fleiss (1972), Everitt (1981) and Grayson (1987)).

1.3.2   History repeating itself: are there two (or more) types of schizophrenia?

One would have thought that, given the lessons learnt from earlier attempts to sub-classify depression, investigators might now have a more sophisticated approach in their attempts to find sub-types of schizophrenia. Such optimism, however, would be misguided. As in the earlier research on depression, a substantial amount of effort has been devoted to attempts to sub-divide schizophrenic patients into distinct groups on the basis of the results of factor analysis of symptom profiles. As in the case of depression, these investigators appear to misunderstand the role and use of factor analysis. Finding that there are apparently two or more dimensions (factors) for psychotic symptoms has no implications one way or the other in terms of whether there might be discrete groups of schizophrenic patients with different aetiology, response to treatment, or long-term prognosis.

Crow (1980) and Andreasen (1982) have postulated the existence of 'positive' and 'negative' sub-types of schizophrenia. This, in turn, has led to the development of standardised assessment scales – the SANS/SAPS (Andreasen, 1983, 1984) and the widespread application of multivariate statistical procedures, such as factor analysis and (more rarely) cluster analysis to investigate patterns of SANS/SAPS symptom scores. The use of factor analysis has confirmed the positive/negative dimensions of schizophrenia, but has also revealed that this two-dimensional view is an oversimplification. We will not go into any further detail here, but refer the interested reader to one of the most recent factor analytic studies (Vázquez-Barquero *et al.*, 1996) in which a four-factor solution was presented. Unlike many of their predecessors, however, these authors did not conclude that there were two (never mind four) discrete types of schizophrenia:

> We have to stress that the demonstration that symptoms ratings can be reduced to summary scores measured on, as it happens in this survey, four different dimensions (four orthogonal factors), does not imply that there are necessarily four distinct subgroups of patients.... The search for evidence of the presence of distinct subgroups of patients belongs to other statistical methods such as, for example, cluster analysis. (Vázquez-Barquero *et al.*, 1996, p. 700).

The results of applying cluster analyses to the patients have been much less consistent or convincing. Van der Does *et al.* (1995), for example, also demonstrated a four-dimensional solution for the symptom correlations. But when they tried several different methods of clustering on their data they admitted that most methods gave a solution in which almost all patients appeared in one large cluster.

Before leaving this section it might be useful to summarise its main message. Whether one is trying to differentiate so-called 'cases' from 'normals', or 'psychotic/endogenous' depressives from 'neurotic/exogenous' depressives, or 'positive' from 'negative' schizophrenics, the split is likely to be entirely arbitrary and artificial. It may, however, be useful. The fact that it is almost essential that we can distinguish 'cases' (who are likely to need help) from the 'non-cases' (who do not) still does not imply that there is some fundamental difference between the two populations. It arises from the introduction of an arbitrary (but useful) boundary between two (or possibly more) regions of a continuum, which, at its simplest might be one-dimensional, but is more likely to have two, three or even more dimensions.

1.4   Study designs

Perhaps the most familiar designs for epidemiological studies in the mental health field are cross-sectional surveys and longitudinal cohort (follow-up) studies, including genetically informative twin and other family studies (see Pickles, 1998, for example). These are the designs that will be referred to the most frequently in the present text. In other areas of epidemiology the case-control study has prominence but this does not appear to be the case in psychiatric epidemiology. One classic example, however, is the investigation of the relationships between life events, social support and depression by Brown and Harris (1978). These authors compared the frequency of putative provoking agents (negative life events, for example), occurring in the presence or absence of vulnerability factors (absence of confiding relationships, for example), in several groups of cases and controls. The three case groups were (1) patients referred to psychiatrists in Camberwell (London, UK) diagnosed as depressed in the absence of alcoholism or other organic causes, (2) an epidemiological case group obtained from two random samples drawn from those living in Camberwell and (3) a group from a rural epidemiological sample. The control group was primarily drawn from non-cases from the two epidemiological Camberwell samples.

The final type of design to be mentioned here is the randomised intervention study and, in particular, the RCT. The first psychiatrist to advocate the use of Fisher's experimental methods in the evaluation of treatments in psychiatry appears to have been Lewis (1946). In his paper he criticises the past use of small series of cases and 'the common lack of co-ordinated plan for the therapeutic experiment'. Of a controlled trial he concludes:

> An organised experiment would demand much that has not hitherto been practicable, including voluntary acceptance of independent hospitals and clinics of an agreed procedure for the selection, management, evaluation

Table 1.1 Recommendations for the design of a clinical trial (from Johnson, 1998)

(i)	Simplification of design through the collection of minimal outcome measures particularly rating scales; select one or two which are the best understood; eliminate any that are proposed because they *might* be useful. Remember that it is better to 'invest in good, careful collection of a small number of variables than measure everything under the sun' (Kraemer *et al.*, 1987).
(ii)	Concentrate effort into obtaining follow-up information on all randomised patients on a few occasions rather than many.
(iii)	Employ a multicentre design to enable entry to a broad range of patients throughout several locations.
(iv)	Use entry criteria which are as broad as possible so that the results can be generalised to a wide population of patients and provide an opportunity to study heterogeneity.
(v)	Forget power calculations since these provide a minimalist approach to sample size determination; aim to recruit at least 100 patients for analysis in *each* treatment group, and preferably 200; a special case should be required in funding applications for using groups of smaller size.
(vi)	Develop a full strategy for complete analysis before the trial database is 'unblinded' to reveal the treatments. This will include definition of separate groups of patients which will be analysed (intention to treat, per protocol); identification of subjects for each analysis; and listing of variables which will be used to produce adjusted analyses for the treatment comparison.
(vii)	Use of recent statistical modelling techniques to enable full and efficient analysis of all available (unbalanced) data rather than restriction to subjects with complete follow-up information.

of mental state, and follow-up investigation of treated, as well as of control cases. Such an experiment, as R.A. Fisher (1942) has demonstrated, requires much forethought and self-discipline on the part of those who carry it out.

Finally, he states that: 'For most important psychiatric conditions, such trials are essential, unless we are prepared to go on taking decades to decide questions which could be settled in a few years.' Such RCTs are now commonplace in psychiatry, whether we are testing a new psychotherapeutic drug or evaluating a novel form of psychotherapy or case management. Readers are referred to one of the many excellent texts on clinical trial methodology for further discussion of the general principles for the design and analysis of RCTs. In particular, they should consult a recent wide-ranging review of the methodological problems for clinical trials in psychiatry by Johnson (1998). Table 1.1 provides a list of Johnson's recommendations concerning the design of a clinical trial. We do not pursue clinical trial methodology to any great extent in this text but we do look at relatively unfamiliar territory in the form of models for compliance– response relationships (see Chapter 7). Recommendation (i) of Table 1.1 cannot be overemphasised. Although the epidemiological studies discussed later in this book may appear to be considerably more complex than an RCT the strength of the modelling techniques described here comes from being very restrained in the choice of the number and type of variables to be recorded. The 'tighter' the design the better. We are **not** advocating collection of all the variables you can think of so that you can subsequently model them using some flashy form of path analysis or structural equations modelling software. Investigations of the latter type are very unconvincing, to say the least.

1.5   The rest of the book

Chapters 2, 3 and 4 concentrate on the statistical evaluation of measuring instruments. Chapter 2 is primarily concerned with *reliability*, whilst Chapters 3 and 4 concentrate more on instrument *validity*. Despite following Rose (1989) and many others in advocating that quantitative data should be analysed and interpreted using methods appropriate to quantitative data, there is an acknowledgement that the case vs. non-case distinction can have utility and Chapter 2, accordingly, spends much time in the discussion of misclassification errors. Chapter 3 introduces *confirmatory factor analysis*. Chapter 5 covers prevalence estimation and the analysis of data to uncover sources of variation in prevalence and, in particular, the analysis of survey designs using *screening questionnaires* subject to misclassification errors.

Chapters 6 and 7 are all in line with our general approach to the analysis and interpretation of data on psychopathology in that all three explicitly deal with data that are (a) quantitative and (b) recognised as being subject to measurement error. They are also frequently multivariate. Most of the statistical methodology can be described under the heading of *covariance structure models* (including confirmatory factor analysis and *structural equation modelling* with *latent variables*). Chapter 6 deals with observational studies – looking at patterns of variation (or stability) over time and also introducing simple ideas of behaviour genetics to study patterns of inheritance. Chapter 7 looks at the problems and challenges of missing data.

Finally, consider recommendation (vii) in Table 1.1: the use of recent statistical modelling techniques to enable full and efficient analysis of all available (unbalanced) data rather than restriction to subjects with complete follow-up information. In the context of an RCT, Johnson is specifically concerned with coping with drop-outs. This topic is discussed briefly in Chapter 7, but this chapter, however, also covers a wider range of situations in which we might have missing observations and discusses ways in which we might cope with them in an effective and efficient manner. One application is in the evaluation of compliance–response relationships. We emphasise here that it is not meant as an alternative to the usual 'intention-to-treat' analysis but as a supplement to the latter that is aimed at furthering our understanding of what might be going on. The reason I finish this chapter on this point, however, is not because of its specific application to trial methodology, but to emphasise the role of relatively sophisticated, but appropriately specified, statistical models throughout the whole range of applications covered by this book.

2

Instrument reliability

2.1 Introduction

In this chapter we consider three questions: (1) what is meant by reliability and how is it measured, (2) what are the implications of less than perfect reliability, and (3) how do we design and analyse studies to evaluate reliability? Most clinicians have an intuitive idea of what the concept of reliability means and that being able to demonstrate that one's measuring instruments have high reliability is a good thing. It is another matter to pin down what is actually meant by the word 'high' (see Shrout, 1998). Reliability concerns the consistency of repeated measurements, where the repetitions might be repeated interviews by the same interviewer, alternative ratings of the same interview (as a video recording) by different raters, alternative forms or repeated administration of a questionnaire, or even different sub-scales of a single questionnaire, and so on. Closely related to the idea of reliability are *precision*, *repeatability*, *reproducibility* and *generalisability*. One learns from elementary texts that reliability is estimated by a correlation coefficient (in the case of a quantitative rating) or a *kappa statistic* (in the case of a qualitative judgement such as a diagnosis). Rarely are clinicians aware of either the formal definition of reliability or of its estimation through the use of various forms of *intraclass correlation coefficient*.

2.2 Product–moment correlation, intraclass correlation and kappa

Before moving on to a more detailed discussion of reliability and its estimation, let us consider a simple example. Table 2.1 shows some data on the measurement of psychological distress obtained through the use of the 12-item version of Goldberg's (1972) General Health Questionnaire (GHQ). A group of clinical psychology students were asked to complete this questionnaire on two occasions, three days apart. On each occasion the sum of the responses of the odd-numbered items was obtained, as was that for the even-numbered

Table 2.1   GHQ scores for 12 clinical psychology students (from Dunn, 1992)

Odd1	Even1	GHQ1	Case1	Odd2	Even2	GHQ2	Case2
7	5	12	1	7	5	12	1
4	4	8	1	4	3	7	1
12	10	22	1	12	12	24	1
5	5	10	1	7	7	14	1
3	7	10	1	3	5	8	1
4	2	6	0	3	1	4	0
3	5	8	1	2	3	5	0
2	2	4	0	3	3	6	0
7	7	14	1	6	8	14	1
3	3	6	0	2	3	5	0
0	2	2	0	3	2	5	0
11	11	22	1	8	8	16	1

Key to variable names:
Odd1 and Odd2 are the sums of the odd items at times 1 and 2, respectively.
Even1 and Even2 are the corresponding sums for the even items.
GHQ1 and GHQ2 are the total scores at times 1 and 2, respectively.
Case1 and Case2 are the corresponding categorisations into case (1) and non-case (0).

items – using Likert scoring for each item. GHQ2 and GHQ1 are the overall totals (GHQ scores) for each of the two occasions. The sub-scale scores for the first occasion are Odd1 and Even1, and those for the second occasion are Odd2 and Even2. In addition to this I have arbitrarily categorised a student as a GHQ 'case' if he or she has a GHQ score greater than 6 – the variable for the two occasions being Case1 and Case2, respectively.

Let us first consider *test–retest reliability* (see Section 2.6) for the total GHQ score. The first thing to do is to look at the data. The simplest way of doing this is using a few graphs. Figure 2.1 shows a plot of GHQ1 against GHQ2. Clearly

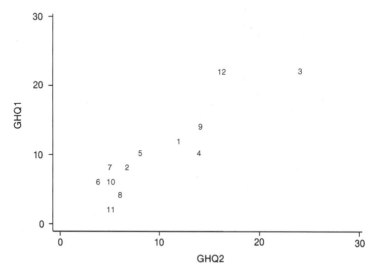

Figure 2.1   Scatter diagram of the GHQ score at time 1 (GHQ1) against the GHQ score at time 2 (GHQ2). The plotting symbol is the subject's identity number (row number in the data as presented in Table 2.1).

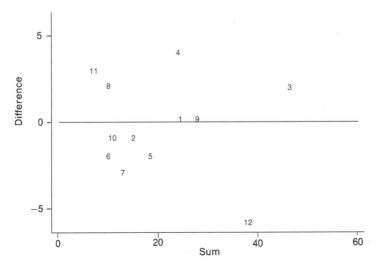

Figure 2.2   Bland–Altman plot for the GHQ data in Table 2.1. The difference (GHQ2 − GHQ1) is plotted against the sum (GHQ2 + GHQ1). A horizontal line is drawn across the plot to indicate a difference of zero. The plotting symbol is the subject's identity number (row number in the data as presented in Table 2.1).

there is a fairly strong association between the two, the product–moment correlation being 0.901. Following suggestions of Bland and Altman (1986) we also plot the difference between the two (i.e. GHQ2 − GHQ1) against their total (GHQ1 + GHQ2). This is shown in Figure 2.2. The disagreements between the two measures do not appear to be related in any systematic way to the overall level. In neither graph does there appear to be any evidence of outlying data points. The mean values for GHQ1 and GHQ2 are 10.33 and 10.00, respectively. The corresponding standard deviations are 6.37 and 6.09.

So, we can estimate the reliability of the GHQ total by a correlation of 0.901. If we use an intraclass correlation coefficient instead, then the reliability is estimated as 0.897. This has been calculated by entering each student's data twice: first with GHQ1 followed by GHQ2 and then by GHQ2 followed by GHQ1 (giving 24 pairs of observations). The product–moment correlation for these 24 pairs of observations is the maximum likelihood estimate of the intraclass (or intrastudent) correlation coefficient (see, for example, Dunn, 1989). This estimator will provide values less than or equal to the product–moment correlation but in many cases their values will be pretty close. In fact, they will only be identical if (a) the observed means of the two sets of scores are the same *and* (b) their observed standard deviations are also identical. An alternative estimator of the intraclass correlation, based on the contents of a one-way analysis of variance (ANOVA) table, is given in Section 2.7 (for the GHQ data, its value turns out to be 0.905).

Cohen's *kappa coefficient* (Cohen, 1960) is a chance-corrected measure of agreement for categorical data. If we look at the agreement between Case1 and Case2 in Table 2.1 we see that the two categorisations agree in 11 out of the 12 students (91.67%). However, if the two categorisations were statistically independent then we would expect 52.78% agreement by chance. The estimate

Table 2.2   Cohen's kappa for diagnostic agreement

Consider the following observed proportions, where n is the total number of patients assessed by two psychiatrists, A and B:

		Psychiatrist A		
		Case	Non-case	Total (marginal proportion)
Psychiatrist B	Case	p_{11}	p_{12}	p_{1+}
	Non-case	p_{21}	p_{22}	p_{2+}
Total (marginal proportion)		p_{+1}	p_{+2}	1

Let $P_o = (p_{11} + p_{22})$ be the observed agreement (measured as a proportion) and $P_c = (p_{1+}p_{+1} + p_{2+}p_{+2})$ be the corresponding chance-expected value. Then kappa (κ) is given by the following expression

$$\kappa = (P_o - P_c)/(1 - P_c)$$

and its sampling variance is

$$\text{var}(\kappa) = (A + B - C)/N(1 - P_c)^4$$

where

$$A = p_{11}[(1 - P_o) - (p_{+1} + p_{1+})(1 - P_o)]^2 + p_{22}[(1 - P_c) - (p_{+2} + p_{2+})(1 - P_o)]^2$$
$$B = (1 - P_o)^2[p_{12}(p_{+1} + p_{2+})^2 + p_{21}(p_{+2} + p_{1+})^2]$$

and

$$C = (P_o P_c - 2P_c + P_o)^2$$

of kappa is 0.824. The Pearson product–moment correlation for binary data (often called a *phi coefficient*) is 0.837. The intraclass correlation (from a one-way ANOVA) is 0.836. They are all fairly close to one another. In fact, if kappa had been calculated assuming that the marginal distributions for Case1 and Case2 were the same (a variant known as Scott's *pi coefficient* – see Scott, 1955), then it is possible to show that for a large sample this kappa is equivalent to the intraclass correlation estimated from a one-way ANOVA. The kappa coefficient itself is asymptotically equivalent to the intraclass correlation estimated from a two-way random effects ANOVA (i.e. Equation 2.3). For this reason, kappa will not be discussed in much detail here (but see Table 2.2). One thing the reader must bear in mind, however, is that significance tests and standard errors obtained throughout the use of a conventional ANOVA are not valid for binary data. Of course, it is fairly straightforward to obtain the required standard errors via bootstrap sampling.

The idea of a chance-corrected measure of agreement can be extended to situations involving more than two observers (see, for example, Fleiss and Cuzick, 1979, or Schouten, 1985), but in this case it becomes even more convenient and straightforward to approach the problem through ANOVA methods. A kappa coefficient for agreement on assessments with more than two categories is a straightforward extension of the binary case (but the ANOVA approach here loses some of its attractions). A weighted version of kappa has also been proposed by Cohen (1968), the weights reflecting differences in the seriousness of the disagreements between raters. For a binary assessment, of course, the unweighted and weighted forms will be the same. The reader is referred to Dunn (1989) for further details.

2.3 Simple measurement models

First consider a quantitative measurement (X). We start with the assumption that it is fallible and that it is the sum of only two components: the 'truth' (T) and 'error' (E). This is the basis of psychometricians' *classical test theory* (Lord and Novick, 1968). If T and E are statistically independent (uncorrelated) then it can be shown that

$$\text{Var}(X) = \text{Var}(T) + \text{Var}(E) \tag{2.1}$$

where $\text{Var}(X)$ is the variance of X (i.e. the square of its standard deviation), and so on. The *coefficient of reliability* of X (R_x) is defined as the proportion of the total variability of X (i.e. $\text{Var}(X)$) that is explained by the variability of the true scores (i.e. $\text{Var}(T)$). That is,

$$R_x = \frac{\text{Var}(T)}{\text{Var}(X)}$$

$$= \frac{\text{Var}(T)}{\text{Var}(T) + \text{Var}(E)} \tag{2.2}$$

R_x is sometimes referred to as a *reliability ratio* and, more often than not, the word 'ratio' is simply dropped. This ratio will approach the value of 0 as the variability of the measurement errors increases in comparison to that of the truth. Alternatively, it will approach 1 as the variability of the errors decreases. The standard deviation of the measurement errors, σ_E (i.e. the square root of $\text{Var}(E)$) is usually known as the instrument's *standard error of measurement*. Note that reliability is not a fixed characteristic of an instrument, even when its standard error of measurement (i.e. its precision) is fixed. When the instrument is used on a population that is relatively homogeneous (relatively low values of $\text{Var}(X)$) it will have a relatively low reliability. On the other hand, as $\text{Var}(T)$ increases then so does the instrument's reliability. In many ways the standard error of measurement is a much more useful summary of an instrument's performance, but one should always bear in mind that it too might vary from one population to another – a possibility that must be carefully checked by both the developers and users of the instrument.

Now let us complicate matters slightly. Suppose that a rating is dependent not only on the subject's so-called true score (T) and random measurement error (E) but also on the identity, say, of the interviewer or rater (I). That is, each interviewer has his or her own characteristic bias (constant from one assessment to another) and that the biases can be thought of as varying randomly from one rater to another. Again, assuming statistical independence, we can show that if $X = T + I + E$, then

$$\text{Var}(X) = \text{Var}(T) + \text{Var}(I) + \text{Var}(E) \tag{2.3}$$

But what is the instrument's reliability? It depends. If subjects in a survey or experiment, for example, are each going to be assessed by a rater randomly selected from a large pool of possible raters, then

$$R_{xa} = \frac{\text{Var}(T)}{\text{Var}(X)}$$

$$= \frac{\text{Var}(T)}{\text{Var}(T) + \text{Var}(I) + \text{Var}(E)} \tag{2.4}$$

But if, on the other hand, only a single rater is to be used for all subjects in the proposed study then there will be no variation due to the rater and the reliability now becomes

$$R_{xb} = \frac{\text{Var}(T)}{\text{Var}(T) + \text{Var}(E)} \tag{2.5}$$

Of course, $R_{xb} > R_{xa}$. Again, the value of the instrument's reliability depends on the context of its use. This is the essence of *generalisability theory* (Cronbach *et al.*, 1972; Shavelson and Webb, 1991). The three versions of R given above are all intraclass correlation coefficients and are also examples of what generalisability theorists refer to as *generalisability coefficients*.

2.4   Implications of measurement error

Suppose that we are interested in estimating the correlation between two quantitative characteristics T_x and T_y but, in fact, we only have observations of fallible measures

$$X = T_x + E_x$$

and

$$Y = T_y + E_y$$

where E_x and E_y are the measurement errors associated with X and Y, respectively. Let the reliabilities of X and Y be R_x and R_y respectively. The true correlation between T_x and T_y is given by

$$\rho_{xy} = \frac{\text{Cov}(T_x, T_y)}{\sqrt{\text{Var}(T_x) \cdot \text{Var}(T_y)}} \tag{2.6}$$

What we actually estimate, however, is

$$\rho'_{xy} = \frac{\text{Cov}(X, Y)}{\sqrt{\text{Var}(X) \cdot \text{Var}(Y)}}$$

$$= \frac{\text{Cov}(T_x + E_x, T_y + E_y)}{\sqrt{\text{Var}(T_x + E_x) \cdot \text{Var}(T_y + E_y)}}$$

$$= \frac{\text{Cov}(T_x, T_y)}{\sqrt{R_x \cdot \text{Var}(T_x) \cdot R_y \cdot \text{Var}(T_y)}}$$

$$= \rho_{xy} \sqrt{R_x \cdot R_y} \tag{2.7}$$

The correlation ρ'_{xy} is subject to *attenuation* (i.e. it shrinks towards 0). The corrected correlation is therefore

$$\rho_{xy} = \frac{\rho'_{xy}}{\sqrt{R_x \cdot R_y}} \tag{2.8}$$

Now consider using a simple least-squares linear regression to predict T_y from a knowledge of T_x. The model is

$$E(T_y | T_x) = \alpha + \beta T_x \tag{2.9}$$

where E( ) denotes expectation, and β is

$$\beta = \frac{\text{Cov}(T_x, T_y)}{\text{Var}(T_x)} \tag{2.10}$$

What we actually estimate from the data is

$$\beta' = \frac{\text{Cov}(X, Y)}{\text{Var}(X)}$$
$$= \frac{R_x \cdot \text{Cov}(T_x, T_y)}{\text{Var}(T_x)}$$
$$= R_x \cdot \beta \tag{2.11}$$

Again, the regression coefficient β' is subject to attenuation (i.e. is shrunk closer to 0) and can be corrected by dividing by the appropriate reliability coefficient, R_x. Note that the reliability of the response (Y) has no relevance here.

In the case of a simple linear logistic regression using a fallible predictor it can also be shown that the estimated regression coefficient (here interpreted as the logarithm of an odds ratio) is attenuated in a qualitatively similar way (see Carroll, Ruppert and Stefanski, 1995, for example). When we are dealing with multiple logistic regression or even with the more familiar multiple linear regression, with one or more covariates (predictors) subject to measurement error then life can be considerably more complicated. Interested readers are referred to Carroll *et al.* (1995) and Fuller (1987) for a detailed discussion.

2.5 More on classical test theory

Starting with the model

$$X = T + E \tag{2.12}$$

and the assumptions concerning the statistical independence of T and E, and also that of Es associated with different measurements (either within or across subjects), we derived

$$\text{Var}(X) = \text{Var}(T) + \text{Var}(E) \tag{2.13}$$

Now,

$$\text{Cov}(X, T) = \text{E}(XT) - \text{E}(X)\text{E}(T)$$
$$= \text{E}[(T + E)T] - \text{E}(T + E)\text{E}(T)$$
$$= \text{E}(T^2) + \text{E}(ET) - \text{E}(T)^2 - \text{E}(E)\text{E}(T)$$
$$= \text{E}(T^2) - \text{E}(T)^2$$
$$= \text{Var}(T) \tag{2.14}$$

Another way of describing the reliability coefficient is, therefore,

$$R_x = \frac{\text{Cov}(X, T)}{\text{Var}(X)} \tag{2.15}$$

This is also equivalent to

$$R_x = \frac{1 - \text{Var}(E)}{\text{Var}(X)} \tag{2.16}$$

It is the proportion of the variability of X that is not due to measurement error.

Now, consider the correlation between the subjects' observed score (X) and the corresponding true score (T):

$$\text{Corr}(X, T) = \frac{\text{Cov}(X, T)}{\sqrt{\text{Var}(X) \cdot \text{Var}(T)}}$$
$$= \frac{\text{Var}(T)}{\sqrt{\text{Var}(X)} \cdot \sqrt{\text{Var}(T)}}$$
$$= \frac{\sqrt{\text{Var}(T)}}{\sqrt{\text{Var}(X)}}$$
$$= \sqrt{R_x} \tag{2.17}$$

If we have two separate instruments providing measurements X and X on each of a sample of subjects, then these instruments are said to be *parallel* if (a) the true scores are the same for the two instruments (i.e. no bias) – T, and (b) the measurement errors for the two instruments have the same variance (i.e. they have the same precision) $\text{Var}(E)$.

So,

$$\text{Var}(X_1) = \text{Var}(T) + \text{Var}(E)$$

and

$$\text{Var}(X_2) = \text{Var}(T) + \text{Var}(E)$$
$$= \text{Var}(X)$$

In addition,

$$\text{Cov}(X_1, X_2) = \text{Var}(T)$$

and, therefore, the correlation between X_1 and X_2 is

$$\text{Corr}(X_1, X_2) = \frac{\text{Cov}(X_1, X_2)}{\sqrt{\text{Var}(X_1) \cdot \text{Var}(X_2)}}$$

$$= \frac{\text{Var}(T)}{\text{Var}(X)}$$

The reliability coefficient is the *correlation between parallel tests*. This is the basis for the estimation of reliability by correlation coefficients as described earlier.

Now consider the reliability of the sum of X_1 and X_2. The true component of the sum is $2T$ with variance $4\text{Var}(T)$. The total is $2T + E_1 + E_2$ with variance $4\text{Var}(T) + 2\text{Var}(E)$. The reliability of $X_1 + X_2$ is therefore given by

$$R_{x_1 + x_2} = \frac{4\text{Var}(T)}{4\text{Var}(T) + 2\text{Var}(E)}$$

$$= \frac{2\text{Var}(T)}{2\text{Var}(T) + \text{Var}(E)}$$

$$= \frac{2\text{Var}(T)}{\text{Var}(X) + \text{Var}(T)}$$

If we now divide both the top and the bottom of this ratio by $\text{Var}(X)$, we obtain

$$R_{x_1 + x_2} = \frac{\dfrac{2\text{Var}(T)}{\text{Var}(X)}}{1 + \dfrac{\text{Var}(T)}{\text{Var}(X)}}$$

$$= \frac{2R_x}{1 + R_x} \qquad (2.18)$$

In general, if we have k parallel tests $(X_1, X_2, \ldots, X_i, \ldots, X_k)$ then the variance of their sum (ΣX_i),

$$\text{Var}(\Sigma X_i) = k^2 \text{Var}(X) + k\text{Var}(E)$$

and

$$\text{Var}(kT) = k^2 \text{Var}(T)$$

Therefore

$$R_{\text{sum}} = \frac{k^2 \text{Var}(T)}{k^2 \text{Var}(X) + k\text{Var}(E)}$$

$$= \frac{k^2 R_x}{k^2 R_x + k(1 - R_x)}$$

$$= \frac{k R_x}{k R_x + (1 - R_x)}$$

$$= \frac{k R_x}{1 + (k - 1)R_x} \qquad (2.19)$$

Equation (2.19) is the well-known *Spearman–Brown prophesy formula*. Let us stop to consider a few simple examples to illustrate the use of this formula. Suppose that the reliability of a score from a single administration of a test is 0.5. And suppose that this is not thought to be high enough. If we were to administer the test twice (with a suitable time interval between the two administrations) what would be the reliability of the average of the two test scores? The answer is given by $2 \times 0.5/(1 + 0.5)$ or 0.67. Now suppose that we have the average of five independent test scores. The reliability of this average is given by $5 \times 0.5/(1 + 4 \times 0.5)$ or 0.83. Finally consider a situation where a single administration of a 50-item test has a reliability of 0.9, for example. If we were to randomly select 25 items from the test and use this, what would be the reliability of the shortened form? This would be given by inserting $\frac{1}{2}$ for k in the Spearman–Brown formula. The required reliability is $\frac{1}{2} \times 0.9/(1 - \frac{1}{2} \times 0.9)$ or 0.82 (if you are not convinced, just work out the reliability of the average of two tests, each with a reliability of 0.82).

2.6   Designs for reliability studies

Table 2.1 illustrates the two most commonly used designs in psychometric test development. The first is simply to take a single measuring device and do a *test–retest reliability study*. If we then assume that there has been no change in the true scores and that test and retest are parallel, then the reliability is estimated by the correlation (or intraclass correlation) between test and retest scores. The second approach depends on the assumption that the constituent items of a test are measuring the same thing. Randomly splitting the items into two equal-sized groups produces a pair of (assumed) parallel tests and hence their correlation estimates their common reliability. The choice of odd and even items in Table 2.1 is not actually a random partition but will be used to illustrate the idea. The product–moment correlation between Odd1 and Even1 is 0.865. The mean and standard deviation of Odd1 are 5.08 and 3.58, respectively. The mean and standard deviation of Even1 are 5.25 and 3.02, respectively. They appear to be more or less parallel. But this *split-half reliability* is the reliability of a test of only six items. What is the reliability of the whole? We now apply the Spearman–Brown formula (Equation 2.19):

$$R_{X_1+X_2} = \frac{2 \times 0.865}{1 + 0.865}$$

$$= 0.928$$

This, of course, is larger than the corresponding test–retest coefficient. They are, however, estimating different things. The test–retest coefficient is a measure of *temporal stability*: in this design random fluctuations in the subjects' true state are indistinguishable from measurement error. The coefficient derived from a split-half correlation is a measure of *internal consistency* (with similar characteristics to the well-known and over-used Cronbach's *alpha coefficient* – see Dunn (1989) or Shrout (1998) for comments on the latter's properties). This distinction can be made transparent by taking a rather extreme example. Suppose we are measuring anxiety by questionnaire – something that is expected to vary quite a lot from day to day. And suppose that we replicate each item in our questionnaire, creating two sub-scales each containing one of the two replicates. We would expect that the split-half correlation would indicate almost perfect internal consistency (which in itself is of no advantage whatsoever – we can easily obtain perfect internal consistency by asking the same question over and over again!) and that the test–retest correlation would be pretty low (which, again, is not very informative since it too is not estimating reliability in the sense that we want it to).

Now consider two simple designs for reliability (generalisability) studies. The first involves each subject of the study being independently assessed by two (or more) raters or interviewers with the raters for any given subject being randomly selected from a very large pool of potential raters. Here raters are said to be *nested within subjects*. The second design again involves each subject of the study being independently assessed by two (or more) raters but in this case the raters are the same for all subjects. Equations (2.1) and (2.2) are relevant to the analysis of data arising from the first design, whilst Equations (2.3), (2.4) and (2.5) are relevant to the analysis of data from the second design.

A variant on the second design which deserves to be used much more often is the *balanced incomplete blocks design (BIBD)* as described by Fleiss (1981, 1987) and Dunn (1989, 1992). The only examples of its use in this area which I am aware of are those described by Fleiss (1987) and by Clare and Cairns (1978). Suppose a study design is chosen in which a fixed panel of psychiatrists is intended to sit in on interviews directed by another clinician. Each psychiatrist simply watches and listens to the interview as a neutral spectator and then independently makes an assessment of the patient's psychiatric condition. This design is satisfactory from many points of view but there is often an important practical constraint imposed which makes it unrealistic. Suppose that the interview room is too small to hold more than three spectators or that the patient and interviewer are incapable of tolerating the presence of more than two spectators. Alternatively, suppose that it is far too expensive and time-consuming for all psychiatrists to attend all interviews.

Obviously, technical devices such as half-silvered mirrors or the use of videotapes can help considerably in this situation. But a further way to cope with the problem is through the use of a BIBD. Another example of a situation in which this type of constraint will be imposed is where each clinician is expected to interview or examine each patient independently. Here, even the most compliant patient is unlikely to tolerate more than two interviews. The use of the BIBD in reliability studies will be illustrated using data in Table 2.3 (from Fleiss, 1981).

Table 2.3 Results of a BIBD reliability study of a rating scale for depression (reproduced with permission from Fleiss, 1981)

Rater	Subject 1	2	3	4	5	6	7	8	9	10
1	10	3	7	3	20					
2	14	3				20	5	14		
3	10		12		14				12	18
4		1		8			8		17	19
5				5	26	20		18	12	
6			9		20		14	15		

Here each of ten subjects is rated for depression by three raters. The study involves a total of six raters and each of these raters assesses five subjects. In the study reported by Clare and Cairns (1978) each of 48 subjects were assessed by two raters. The study involved the use of a total of four raters and each of these raters assessed 24 subjects. Each distinct pair of raters jointly rated eight subjects. Further technical details of the design can be found elsewhere (Fleiss, 1987; Dunn, 1989).

2.7   Estimation of reliability from ANOVA tables

When we come to analyse the data it is usually appropriate to carry out an *analysis of variance (ANOVA)*. For the first design we carry out a *one-way ANOVA* (*X* by subject) and for the second one a *two-way ANOVA* (*X* by rater by subject). In the latter case we assume that there are no subject by rater interactions and constrain the corresponding sum of squares to be 0 accordingly. We assume that readers are reasonably familiar with an analysis of variance table. Each subject has been assessed by, say, k interviewers. The one-way ANOVA yields a mean square for between-subjects variation (BMS) and a mean square for within-subjects variation (WMS). WMS is an estimate of $\text{Var}(E)$ in Equation (2.1). The square root of WMS therefore provides an estimate of the instrument's standard error of measurement. The corresponding estimate of R_x is given by

$$R_x = \frac{BMS - WMS}{BMS + (k-1)WMS} \tag{2.20}$$

In the case of $k = 2$, R_x becomes

$$R_x = \frac{BMS - WMS}{BMS + WMS} \tag{2.21}$$

Moving on to the slightly more complex two-way ANOVA, the ANOVA table provides values of mean squares for subjects – or patients (PMS), interviewers (IMS) and error (EMS). We will not concentrate on the details of estimation of the components of Equation (2.3) – see Dunn (1989), Fleiss (1987) or Streiner and Norman (1995) – but simply note that R_{xa} is estimated by

$$R_{xa} = \frac{n(PMS - EMS)}{n \cdot PMS + k \cdot IMS + (nk - n - k)EMS} \tag{2.22}$$

where the dots indicate multiplication and n is the number of subjects (patients) in the study. Where a single rater or interviewer is to make all the assessments, then

$$R_{xb} = \frac{PMS - EMS}{PMS + (k-1)EMS} \tag{2.23}$$

In reporting the results of a reliability study it is important that the investigators give some idea of the precision of their estimates of reliability, for example, by giving an appropriate standard error, or even better, an

Table 2.4   ANOVA results for GHQ data

(a) One-way ANOVA

Source of variation	S.S.	d.f.	Mean square
Students	811.333	11	73.758
Residual	44.000	12	3.667

$$R_x = (73.758 - 3.667)/(73.758 + 3.667)$$
$$= 0.905$$

(b) Two-way ANOVA

Source of variation	S.S.	d.f.	Mean square
Students	811.333	11	73.758
Time	0.667	1	0.667
Error	43.333	11	3.939

$$R_{xa} = 12(73.758 - 3.939)/[12(73.758) + 2(0.667) + 10(3.939)]$$
$$= 0.905$$
$$R_{xb} = (73.758 - 3.939)/(73.758 + 3.939)$$
$$= 0.899$$

appropriate confidence interval. The subject is beyond the scope of this chapter, however, and the interested reader is referred to Fleiss (1987) or Dunn (1989) for further illumination.

Table 2.4 presents two ANOVAs for the GHQ totals given in Table 2.1. Part (a) gives the one-way ANOVA (GHQ by student – assuming that there are no time trends), and Part (b) gives the corresponding two-way ANOVA (GHQ by time by student). In this particular example it makes little or no difference what model is used – there is no time effect to influence the estimates.

It might be of some interest to the reader to see what happens if we artificially introduce a time effect by adding 5 to all of the GHQ2 scores. In the one-way ANOVA the student mean square remains the same (as expected) but the residual mean square rises to 14.5. The estimate of reliability has now dropped accordingly to 0.803 (note that the product–moment correlation is not affected by constants being added to GHQ2). In the two-way ANOVA the student and error mean squares remain the same but the time mean square is now 130.667. R_{xa} is now 0.707. R_{xb} is unchanged – it is, of course, equivalent to the product–moment correlation.

Details of the ANOVA calculations for the BIBD data in Table 2.2 are provided by Fleiss (1987) – they are beyond the scope of this text. With designs such as this, however (and in other designs involving missing data either by design or happenstance), maximum likelihood (ML) estimation or residual maximum likelihood (REML) estimation should be given serious consideration. These could be obtained through the use of *variance components* or *multilevel modelling* software. Although multilevel modelling is the province of specialist statistical packages, variance components programs are available in many of the general-purpose software packages. Fleiss's ANOVA estimate of the reliability of the depression scores was 0.78 – treating raters as a fixed effect. The REML estimate given by Dunn (1992) is identical. Treating raters as random effects, the REML estimate is 0.79 (the rater effects are very small).

3

Instrument validity

3.1 Introduction

An instrument's *validity* is an indicator of how well it is measuring the characteristic or property it is supposed to measure. Traditionally, the validity of an instrument has been described in three ways (Carmines and Zeller, 1979). *Content validity* refers to the meaning and coverage of the items in a questionnaire or structured interview, for example. *Criterion-related validity* (either *concurrent* or *predictive*) is evaluated by comparing measurements with some sort of external criterion or *gold standard*). Finally, *construct validity* is evaluated by investigating in detail what characteristics an instrument appears to be measuring. The evaluation of content and construct validity are substantive or scientific issues than statistical ones – but are related to some of the ideas concerning covariance structures to be discussed in Chapter 4. Here we will be primarily concerned with criterion-related validity. In particular, we will be concerned with the ability of a screening questionnaire to correctly identify (or rule out) a case of mental illness as determined by a structured or semi-structured diagnostic interview. We are looking at *misclassification errors* as opposed to errors that may be **solely** to do with the measurement process. The performance of a screening instrument may be poor (in terms of misclassification errors) either because it is imprecise (unreliable) or because it is measuring something different to the criterion (gold standard) or **both**. Obviously imprecision affects the performance of a screening questionnaire but even a perfectly precise instrument is likely to make classification errors. On the other hand, there is a limit to an instrument's validity that is determined by its reliability (see, for example, Equation (2.7)). This issue has been explored in the context of the validity of screening questionnaires such as the GHQ by Shrout and Fleiss (1981) and by Goldberg and Williams (1988).

The *sensitivity* of a screening instrument (or screen, for short) is defined as the probability of the screen providing a positive result given that mental illness is present. The *specificity* of the screen is the probability of the screen providing a negative outcome given that mental illness is absent. These and other related

Table 3.1   Characteristics of screening questionnaires

(a) Counts

		True diagnosis (outcome of interview)		
		Positive	Negative	Total
	Positive	a	b	$a+b$
Screen result	Negative	c	d	$c+d$
	Total	$a+c$	$b+d$	$N = a+b+c+d$

(b) Definitions

In terms of the counts a (number of true positives), b (false positives), c (false negatives) and d (true negatives):

Sensitivity (se)	$= a/(a+c)$
Specificity (sp)	$= d/(b+d)$
Positive predictive value (PPV)	$= a/(a+b)$
Negative predictive value (NPV)	$= d/(c+d)$
Likelihood ratio (LR)	$= \text{Sensitivity}/(1 - \text{Specificity})$

characteristics of screening tests are defined in Table 3.1. Here we concentrate on sensitivity and specificity. Estimation of sensitivity and specificity (together with their binomial standard errors) is very straightforward provided one has a simple random sample of subjects, each of which provides a screen result and an independent psychiatric diagnosis. In practice, however, such a sample is rarely available. Whether by design, or by happenstance, there are likely to be *verification biases*. Typically, each subject will first complete a screening questionnaire. Some time later the subject then takes part in a structured or semi-structured psychiatric interview. For example, each member of a large community survey sample might be asked to complete the GHQ. On the basis of the questionnaire results the subjects are then stratified into either GHQ-positives or GHQ-negatives. Further samples are then drawn from each of these two strata for further investigation using, for example, the Clinical Interview Schedule (Goldberg *et al.*, 1970) – the revised version, abbreviated to CIS-R (see Lewis *et al.*, 1992). Typically, most if not all of the GHQ-positives will be interviewed but perhaps only 10–30% of the GHQ-negatives. Finally, the interviewer classifies the members of these sub-samples as diagnosis positive or negative, leading to the familiar cross-classification of the second-phase sub-sample. The two stages of sampling are an example of *double* (or *two-phase*) sampling. Double samples are quite common in psychiatric epidemiology and their analysis will be covered in some detail in later chapters, but in the present chapter we will limit the discussion of them to the purpose of screen validation.

But what of other forms of verification bias? It is not unusual for a subject to refuse to co-operate in a psychiatric interview or, for one reason or another not linked to the formal design, be lost from the study after the results of the initial screen are known but before the diagnostic interview has been carried out. If the refusals or dropouts were to occur completely at random then this would not affect the results (other than simply reducing the final sample size). If the dropouts were not completely random, however, but were related to the psychiatric state or social and demographic characteristics of the subject, then this would lead to biased estimates. The way of dealing with this problem (in this situation, at least) is exactly the same as if the missing data were by design (i.e. through the use of *sampling weights*) and so it will not be explicitly dealt with in any detail below (but see Chapters 5 and 7 for further discussion of this issue).

3.2 Double sampling using screening questionnaires

Prospective sampling simply implies that the investigator obtains a sample of screen-positive patients and a similar sample of screen-negatives, and then ascertains their true diagnosis in order to validate the initial screening. The paper by Bush *et al.* (1987) is an example of a study to validate the use of a simple screening test – using the CAGE Questionnaire (see Ewing, 1984) – to detect alcohol dependence and/or alcohol abuse. The CAGE Questionnaire simply comprises the following four questions:

1. Have you felt the need to Cut down drinking?
2. Have you ever felt Annoyed by criticism of drinking?
3. Have you had Guilty feelings about drinking?
4. Do you ever take a morning Eye-opener?

Bush *et al.* carried out a prospective study of 518 patients admitted to the ortho-paedic and medical services of a community-based teaching hospital during a six-month period. All patients answered the CAGE questions. Diagnostic inter-views were then performed on all 142 of the CAGE-positive patients (those answering 'Yes' to one or more of the screening questions) and a consecutive sub-sample (102 of 376) of the CAGE-negative patients. Following the diagnos-tic interview the investigators classified the second-phase patients as 'normal', 'alcohol abusers' or 'alcohol dependent' (the latter category clearly also includes the second one, but not vice versa). Here we will restrict the discussion to the detection of alcohol abuse. The data are shown in Table 3.2. Of the 142 CAGE-positives, 99 abused alcohol (a PPV of $99/142 = 69.7\%$). Of the 102 interviewed CAGE-negatives, only five were subsequently found to be alcohol abusers (an NPV of $97/102 = 95.1\%$). The overall proportion of CAGE-positives (that is $P(\text{Screen}+)$) is $142/518$ or 27.4%. The standard errors and confidence intervals of each of these three probabilities are quite straightforward as they are all binomial. To estimate the sensitivity and specificity of the CAGE we could use *Bayes' theorem* but here we chose to illustrate the use of *sampling* or *expansion weights* instead. These are often also called *probability weights*.

The analysis is restricted to only those subjects with complete (i.e. second-phase) data. The sampling weight is simply the reciprocal of the second-phase sampling fraction. Using the CAGE data from Table 3.2, the sampling fraction (f_1) for the CAGE-positives is 1 and, therefore, so is the corresponding expan-sion weight (w_1). The second-phase sampling fraction for the CAGE-negatives (f_2), however, is $102/376$ and therefore the corresponding expansion weight

Table 3.2 Characteristics of the CAGE (Bush *et al.*, 1987)

(a) First-phase sample

CAGE-positive	142
CAGE-negative	376
Total	518
P (Screen-positive)	142/518 or 27.4%

(b) Second-phase sample

		Alcohol abuse		
		Positive	Negative	Total
The CAGE	Positive	$a = 99$	$b = 43$	$a + b = 142$
	Negative	$c = 5$	$d = 97$	$c + d = 102$

$$PPV = 99/142 \text{ or } 69.7\%$$

$$NPV = 97/102 \text{ or } 95.1\%$$

(w_2) is 376/102. The sampling weight is an indicator of how many of the original phase-one sample is 'represented by' data from each of the second-phase participants.

In general, in our calculations of sensitivity and specificity, instead of the simple fractions given in Table 3.1, we replace a by aw_1, b by bw_1, c by cw_2 and d by dw_2.

So,

$$\text{Sensitivity} = \frac{aw_1}{aw_1 + cw_2} \tag{3.1}$$

$$= \frac{99}{99 + (5 \times 376/102)}$$

$$= 0.843$$

$$\text{Specificity} = \frac{dw_2}{bw_1 + dw_2} \tag{3.2}$$

$$= \frac{(97 \times 376/102)}{(97 \times 376/102) + 43}$$

$$= 0.893$$

Note that one characteristic of the prospective two-phase design is that if the calculation is performed in the same way for the PPV and NPV the weights simply cancel out. There is no need to use sampling weights in the calculation of the PPV or the NPV (Tarnoplosky *et al.*, 1979). Another way of thinking of these weighted estimates is from the point of view of expansion weights for each of the individual subjects' observation. Individual *i* has an associated weight w_i (which is the reciprocal of its corresponding cell sampling fraction). In the present example, all the CAGE-positives have a weight of 1; that for each of the CAGE-negatives is 3.686 (the reciprocal of 102/376). Considering the estimation of specificity, for example, this is equivalent to

$$\text{Specificity} = \frac{\Sigma_i y_i w_i}{\Sigma_i w_i} \qquad (3.3)$$

where $y_i = 1$ for a true negative and $y_i = 0$ for a false one. This is an example of a *Horvitz–Thompson estimator* (Lehtonen and Pahkinen, 1995; Särndal *et al.*, 1992). One of the advantages of this estimator is that it leads to a reasonably straightforward method for the estimation of its standard error. Its variance can be estimated using the *delta technique* (see Appendix 3 of Dunn, 1989). For two random variables, A and B, the variance of the ratio $R = A/B$ is given by

$$\text{Var}(R) = R^2 \left[\frac{\text{Var}(A)}{A^2} + \frac{\text{Var}(B)}{B^2} - \frac{2\text{Cov}(A, B)}{AB} \right] \qquad (3.4)$$

We use straightforward calculations to determine the variance of the product $y_i w_i$ (2.912), the variance of w_i (1.546) and their covariance (2.122). To go to the variance and covariance for the totals we simply multiply by the number of CAGE-negatives tested (102). The mean of $y_i w_i$ is 2.554, and that for w_i is 2.861. The ratio of these two means (equivalent to the ratio of the two totals in expression (2.17)) is 0.893, the required specificity estimate. Plugging all of these values into Equation (3.4) leads to a variance estimate of 0.000311. The required standard error for the specificity is the square root of this variance (i.e. 0.0178).

Table 3.3 illustrates the second-phase results of a survey of psychiatric morbidity from Verona in northern Italy (Picinelli *et al.*, 1995). In the first phase 1558 participants were asked to complete the GHQ-12. These subjects were then stratified according to their GHQ score (low, medium or high) and sub-samples of these three strata were then interviewed using the Composite International Diagnostic Interview – Primary Care Version, the CIDI-PHC (see Von Korff and Üstün, 1995). Let us arbitrarily pick a GHQ score cut-off of between 6 and 7 in order to classify subjects as possible cases (or not) according to the GHQ. The weighted estimates of sensitivity and specificity are 0.18 and 0.96, respectively. Instead of using Equation (3.4) to estimate their standard errors, we will consider the derivation of a 95% confidence interval. If the estimated point estimates of the sensitivities and specificities are reasonably close to 1 then a symmetrical confidence interval is unlikely to be particularly realistic. Here it is perhaps more appropriate (and often more convenient) to carry out a weighted logistic regression (which will not be considered in detail here – see Chapter 5) on the true positives and the true negatives, separately, in order to obtain a confidence interval for the logits of the sensitivity and specificity. Taking the true positives, for example, and considering the probability of being a screen-positive, one can estimate the logit of this probability by simply fitting a constant to the data. This logit can be assumed to be normally distributed with an estimated standard error provided by appropriate logistic regression software. A 95% confidence interval for this logit is then given by the point estimate plus or minus 1.96 standard errors. The inverse of the logistic transformation then provides the confidence interval for the probability itself. A similar analysis can be carried out for the true negatives – but here modelling

Table 3.3   Second-phase data from Verona: GHQ score by CIDI-PHC case (Piccinelli *et al.*, 1995)

		Interview result	
		Non-case	Case
Stratum 1 (weight = 17.48)			
GHQ score	0	20	8
	1	5	7
	2	4	5
	3	4	7
Stratum 2 (weight = 4.94)			
GHQ score	4	10	21
	5	4	13
Stratum 3 (weight = 1.92)			
GHQ score	6	8	37
	7	7	26
	8	5	20
	9	2	20
	10	1	6
	11	0	6
	12	0	4

Characteristics of the GHQ using a cut-off of 6/7

$$\text{Sensitivity} = \frac{82 \times 1.92}{(27 \times 17.48) + (34 \times 4.94) + (119 \times 1.92)}$$

$$= 0.18$$

$$\text{Specificity} = \frac{(33 \times 17.48) + (14 \times 4.94) + (8 \times 1.92)}{(33 \times 17.48) + (14 \times 4.94) + (23 \times 1.92)}$$

$$= 0.96$$

the probability of being a screen-negative. Returning to the Verona survey, using the logit command within *Stata* (StataCorp, 1997) (together with appropriate sampling weights), we obtain 95% confidence intervals of $(0.14, 0.24)$ and $(0.93, 0.98)$ for sensitivity and specificity, respectively.

3.3   Quantitative test results: ROC curves

In most circumstances the diagnostic test or screening questionnaire yields a score rather than a binary $(+/-)$ result. It is only for convenience that a cut-off is used to classify respondents into test positives and test negatives. The Verona data in Table 3.3 clearly illustrate that, if the purpose of the screening questionnaire is to provide a means of stratification in a two-phase survey, then there is no need to arbitrarily divide the first-phase sample into so-called 'cases' and 'non-cases'. Picinelli *et al.* (1995) chose to use three first-phase strata instead of the more usual two. However, there are often situations

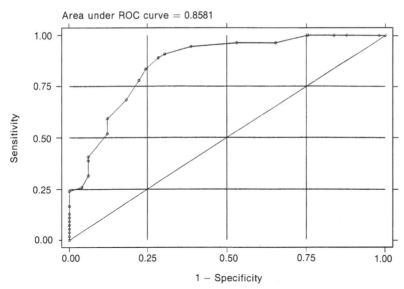

Figure 3.1 A receiver operating characteristic curve for the HADS (data from Lewis *et al.*, 1992).

where one might wish to evaluate the effects of different cut-offs even after collecting the data using a particular two-phase design. The choice of the best cut-off is often determined through the use of a *receiver operating characteristic* (*ROC*) curve (see, for example, Hanley and McNeill, 1982). Here the cut-off is varied throughout the whole range of possibilities and the sensitivity and specificity estimated for each of the cut-off values. The ROC curve is then a plot of sensitivity against 1 − specificity (that is, the true positive rate against the false positive rate). A test which cannot discriminate between cases and non-cases (i.e. when sensitivity = 1 − specificity for all choices of cut-off) produces a straight line with unit slope. A good discriminator produces a curve that concentrates in the upper left corner of the graph. The production of ROC curves from data arising from simple random sampling without verification biases is straightforward but in the case of data arising from prospective two-phase sampling one needs to remember to use expansion weights in the estimation of the appropriate sensitivities and specificities. Figure 3.1 illustrates a ROC curve for the Hospital Anxiety and Depression Scale – the HADS (Zigmond and Snaith, 1983) using data described in Lewis *et al.* (1992). The raw data are given in Table 3.4. A reasonable cut-off appears to be around 11/12.

A similar procedure (remembering to use weighted counts) could be used for the second-phase data from the Verona survey in Table 3.3. One way of assessing the utility of a screening questionnaire is to estimate the area under the ROC curve (or *area under the curve* – *AUC*). The AUC is the probability that a randomly selected case will score higher on the screening questionnaire than a randomly selected non-case (Hanley and McNeill, 1982). For the HADS (using the data of Lewis *et al.*) it is 0.86. The AUC can be estimated

Table 3.4 Scores from the Hospital Anxiety and Depression Scale (HADS) (from Lewis *et al.*, 1992)

HADS	Counts		Test characteristics*		
	CIS-R negative	CIS-R positive	se(%)	sp(%)	1 − sp(%)
0	1	0	100	0	100
1	5	0	100	2	98
2	2	0	100	12	88
3	4	0	100	16	84
4	5	2	100	24	76
5	6	1	96	35	65
6	7	1	95	47	53
7	4	2	93	61	39
8	1	1	89	69	31
9	2	3	87	71	29
10	1	3	82	76	24
11	2	5	76	78	22
12	3	5	67	82	18
13	0	4	58	88	12
14	3	6	51	88	12
15	0	1	40	94	6
16	0	4	38	94	6
17	1	3	31	94	6
18	2	1	25	96	4
19	0	0	24	100	0
20	0	4	24	100	0
21	0	2	16	100	0
22	0	0	13	100	0
23	0	1	13	100	0
24	0	1	11	100	0
25	0	0	9	100	0
26	0	0	9	100	0
27	0	1	9	100	0
28	0	1	7	100	0
29	0	1	5	100	0
30	0	1	4	100	0
31	0	0	4	100	0
32	0	0	4	100	0
33	0	0	4	100	0
34	0	0	4	100	0
35	0	1	2	100	0
Total	49	55			

* Cut-off 1 below current HADS score

from the ROC plot directly (using the trapezoid rule) or it can be approached from a different direction. The numerator for an AUC estimate is the number of case/non-case pairs in which the screen is higher in the case than in the non-case (i.e. the *Mann–Whitney U statistic*). The denominator is the total number of possible case/non-case pairs in the whole sample. In the case of verification biases (e.g. in two-phase sampling) we calculate the same numerator and denominator but after first using sampling weights to get a weighted estimate of these counts. In summary, the AUC in the case of verification biases is simply the weighted Mann–Whitney U statistic divided by the weighted estimate of the number of possible case/non-case pairs. Standard errors can be estimated through the use of the delta technique or bootstrap sampling.

Zhou (1996) has derived the above estimator as the non-parametric maximum likelihood estimator of the AUC. Further details, including a discussion of appropriate software, can be found in Zhou (1998).

3.4 Comparison of screening methods

Table 3.5 shows the result of a two-phase survey from Cantabria in northern Spain (Vázquez-Barquero *et al.*, 1997). In the first phase of the survey the

Table 3.5 Second-phase data from Cantabria: screen status by SCAN case (from Vázquez-Barquero *et al.*, 1997)

(a) Basic data	SCAN result	
	Non-case	Case
Stratum 1 (weight = 12.24)		
GHQ-negative and GP-negative	34	8
Stratum 2 (weight = 1.92)		
GHQ-positive and GP-negative	48	41
GHQ-negative and GP-positive	10	7
GHQ-positive and GP-positive	19	36

(b) Re-arranged SCAN cases (weighted total = 259)

		GP status	
		Negative	Positive
	Negative	8 × 12.24 (= 97.92)	7 × 1.92 (= 13.44)
GHQ status			
	Positive	41 × 1.92 (= 78.72)	36 × 1.92 (= 69.12)

GHQ sensitivity   = 57%

GP sensitivity   = 32%

Screen sensitivity = 62%

(c) Re-arranged SCAN non-cases (weighted total = 564)

		GP status	
		Negative	Positive
	Negative	34 × 12.24 (= 416.16)	10 × 1.92 (= 19.20)
GHQ status			
	Positive	48 × 1.92 (= 92.16)	19 × 1.92 (= 36.48)

GHQ specificity   = 77%

GP specificity   = 90%

Screen specificity = 74%

subjects were independently screened in two ways: the mental health status of the patients was determined through information provided by the general practitioner (GP) and the GHQ-28 (Goldberg and Williams, 1988). Patients were independently classified as being either GP-positive (a case identified by the GP) or GP-negative, and as GHQ-positive (a case identified by the GHQ using a score of 5 or more) or GHQ-negative. The screen-positives were defined by patients being GP-positive or GHQ-positive, or both; otherwise they were screen-negatives. Second-phase patients were then sub-sampled from these two strata (as defined by screen status) and given a detailed psychiatric interview using the SCAN (Wing *et al.*, 1990). As well as providing the phase-two counts, Table 3.5 illustrates further the estimation of sensitivities and specificities. In this example, however, the calculations can be applied to the GP, the GHQ and also the composite screen. The GHQ has a sensitivity that is quite a lot higher than that for the GP. As expected from its definition, the composite screen has an even higher sensitivity, but not much so. On the other hand, the GP is much more specific than the GHQ. Comparison of the sensitivities, say, of the GHQ and GP, can be carried out using the marginal logistic regression models to be described in Chapter 5 (the resulting χ^2 statistic based on the square of the ratio of the appropriate regression coefficient to its robust standard error is 20.78 with one degree of freedom). One could, however, use a simple McNemar test for the comparison of two correlated proportions: $\chi^2 = (41 - 7)^2/(41 + 7) = 20.08$ with one degree of freedom ($P \ll 0.05$).

We will not go into details here, but another, in many ways preferable, approach to the comparison of screening questionnaires and diagnostic tests (unless they really do have binary outcomes) is through the comparison of the AUC estimates from their ROC curves (see Zhou, 1998, for example). Simple bootstrap methods could easily be implemented for this purpose.

3.5   Implications of classification errors

Consider a survey in which the only source of information concerning the presence of mental illness is a classification into 'case' or 'non-case' according to the GHQ. Suppose that we are interested in the comparison of the prevalence of disorder in men and women. Let the true prevalence of psychiatric disorder in men and women be π_m and π_f, respectively. So we are interested, say, in the arithmetic difference $\pi_m - \pi_f$. What we actually estimate is $P_m - P_f$ where P_m and P_f are the true proportions of GHQ-positives in men and women, respectively.

Let the sensitivity of the GHQ for males be represented by $(1 - \delta_m)$ and that for females be $(1 - \delta_f)$. Similarly, let the corresponding specificities for males and females be $(1 - \phi_m)$ and $(1 - \phi_f)$, respectively. It follows that:

$$P_m = \pi_m(1 - \delta_m) + (1 - \pi_m)\phi_m \tag{3.5}$$

and

$$P_f = \pi_f(1 - \delta_f) + (1 - \pi_f)\phi_f \tag{3.6}$$

Therefore

$$P_m - P_f = \pi_m(1 - \delta_m) + (1 - \pi_m)\phi_m - \pi_f(1 - \delta_f) - (1 - \pi_f)\phi_f$$

$$= (\pi_m - \pi_f) + (\phi_m - \phi_f) + \pi_f(\delta_f + \phi_f) - \pi_m(\delta_m + \phi_m) \quad (3.7)$$

$P_m - P_f$ is typically a biased estimator of the difference $(\pi_m - \pi_f)$. In fact, the estimated difference might be less than $(\pi_m - \pi_f)$, or equal to it, or even greater. It may even be of the opposite sign! We might be prepared to make simplifying assumptions, however. If the sensitivities in the two groups are the same (i.e. $\delta_m = \delta_f = \delta$, say) and the specificities are also equal (i.e., $\phi_m = \phi_f = \phi$, say), then it follows that

$$P_m - P_f = (\pi_m - \pi_f) + \pi_f(\delta + \phi) - \pi_m(\delta + \phi)$$

$$= (\pi_m - \pi_f) + (\pi_f - \pi_m)(\delta + \phi)$$

$$= (\pi_m - \pi_f)(1 - \delta - \phi) \quad (3.8)$$

Notice that Equation (3.8) implies that unless δ and ϕ are both equal to zero, $P_m - P_f$ cannot be equal to $\pi_m - \pi_f$. As long as both δ and ϕ are *both* less than 0.5 there cannot be a sign reversal. $P_m - P_f$ will, however, be closer to zero than $\pi_m - \pi_f$.

3.6   Variation in validity coefficients

Clearly there is a need to examine the validity of screening questionnaires for different social and demographic groups. It is neither safe nor justified to assume that the sensitivities and specificities are homogeneous. Table 3.6

Table 3.6   Sex differences in the sensitivity and specificity of the GHQ-60[**] with respect to case definition defined by the Present State Examination (Vázquez-Barquero *et al.*, 1986)

Psychiatric cases

	Males			Females		
	Count (C)	Weight[*] (W)	W × C	Count (C)	Weight[*] (W)	W × C
GHQ+	21	68/68	21.00	85	159/151	89.50
GHQ−	5	513/109	23.53	11	483/124	42.85
Total			44.53			132.35
	Sensitivity = 47%			Sensitivity = 68%		

Normals

	Males			Females		
	Count (C)	Weight* (W)	W × C	Count (C)	Weight* (W)	W × C
GHQ+	46	68/68	46.00	68	159/151	71.60
GHQ−	106	513/109	498.88	110	483/124	428.47
Total			544.88			500.07
	Specificity = 92%			Specificity = 86%		

[*] Number of phase-one subjects/number of phase-two subjects
[**] Using an 11/12 threshold

illustrates calculations for data comparing the GHQ-60 and the Present State Examination (Wing *et al.*, 1974) in a survey undertaken by Vázquez-Barquero *et al.* (1986). The GHQ appears to be more sensitive in females but, as might be expected, less specific – but the differences in specificity are minor. Other direct comparisons of the validity coefficients for men and women (reported in Goldberg and Williams, 1988) tend to confirm this picture; the sensitivity tends to be lower in males (on average 64% in men versus 80% in women) but specificity is about the same (about 85%).

If one chooses to model the variation of validity coefficients using techniques such as logistic models one needs to bear in mind the following questions:

(a) How have the data been collected?
(b) Are we modelling sensitivity/specificity or predictive values?

If the answer to (a) is that we have a simple random sample of participants in which everyone provides a result for the screen and the criterion then there is no need to bother about verification biases and the corresponding sampling weights. If the answer to (a) is that we have a prospective two-phase study with screen used at phase one and criterion at phase two then we have to think carefully about the use of sampling weights in our models (see Chapter 5). As in the case of simple estimation problems, weights are required for the valid modelling of sensitivity and specificity. They are not required, however, if we are modelling predictive values (the PPV or NPV).

Under certain circumstances the answer to question (a) might be that a two-phase design was used but that it was *retrospective* in the following sense (Kraemer, 1992). Everyone in the first-phase sample provides information on whether they are ill or not (as determined by the gold standard). These participants are then stratified into cases and non-cases with the phase-two sample being drawn from these strata with (possibly) unequal sampling fractions. These are sometimes called *case-control* designs. Retrospective designs are often used in the evaluation of laboratory tests. A first-phase sample of depressed patients might be obtained and classified into two: those patients, say, suffering from endogenous depression (melancholia) versus those suffering from neurotic or exogenous depression. Subsamples (phase two) of these two classes might then be given a laboratory test – the dexamethasone suppression test (DST), for example: see Carroll *et al.* (1982) – and their test results classified as positive or negative. In this situation the estimates of sensitivity and specificity (with respect to the detection of endogenous depression) would **not** be weighted but those of predictive values would need appropriate sampling weights. The same would apply to logistic regression models.

3.7   Latent class models

In this section we assume that the reader is familiar with log-linear models for contingency tables (see Everitt and Dunn, 1991) and use them to test hypotheses concerning associations in a multiway table of cases defined by three or more methods of case definition. The section is technically more demanding than the rest of the chapter but this should not put the reader off. It is included to give the reader some idea of what might be done once we relax the assumption that the psychiatrist's decision is not subject to misclassification errors.

Table 3.7   Cross-classification of caseness defined by the GHQ, the HADS and the CIS-R (data from the study of Lewis *et al.*, 1992)

CIS-R ($h = 1, 2$)	GHQ ($i = 1, 2$)	HADS ($j = 1, 2$)	Count (n_{hij})
1	1	1	35
1	1	2	5
1	2	1	3
1	2	2	6
2	1	1	6
2	1	2	8
2	2	1	6
2	2	2	34

Key: 1 = non-case; 2 = case

Returning to the data of Lewis *et al.* (1992), if the case definition provided by the CIS-R were error-free **and** if the association between the results of screening by the GHQ and HADS only arose because they were measuring caseness as defined by the CIS-R, then this would imply that the GHQ and the HADS should be statistically-independent, conditional on true status. This property is often referred to as *local independence*. Table 3.7 shows the three-way contingency table for these data. Fitting a log-linear model to these counts with the following form:

$$\log(m_{hij}) = \text{CONST} + \text{CIS-R}(h) + \text{GHQ}(i) + \text{HADS}(j)$$
$$+ \text{CIS-R}(h).\text{GHQ}(i) + \text{CIS-R}(h).\text{HADS}(j) \qquad (3.9)$$

where m_{hij} is the fitted value corresponding to the observed count n_{hij}, and with the usual parameter constraints for identifiability (see Everitt and Dunn, 1991, for example), provides a test of the conditional independence hypothesis. The resulting likelihood-ratio chi-square (deviance) is 14.859 with two degrees of freedom. Obviously the conditional independence assumption does not hold.

To cope with this problem we change tack. Let us accept that the use of the CIS-R is subject to misclassification errors. This would mean that in any statistical model the three methods of case definition would be treated symmetrically. An implication of this change is that there is a *latent* or *hidden class*, which represents some sort of consensus between the three methods. It might be tempting to regard this latent class as the 'truth', but this would be mistaken. It is simply a classification that maximises the agreement between the three methods, defined in terms of the local independence assumption. This assumption now takes the form of postulating that any two observed indicators of caseness are statistically independent given the identity of the latent class (consensus). In terms of a log-linear model for the resulting four-way contingency table, it implies the following:

$$\log(m_{hijk}) = \text{CONST} + \text{CIS-R}(h) + \text{GHQ}(i) + \text{HADS}(j) + \text{LC}(k)$$
$$+ \text{CIS-R}(h).\text{LC}(k) + \text{GHQ}(i).\text{LC}(k) + \text{HADS}(j).\text{LC}(k) \quad (3.10)$$

where $\text{LC}(k = 1, 2)$ is the postulated latent class. The problem, of course, is that LC is not observed. Using the symbol '+' to indicate a marginal count, the table we observe is a three-way table of the N_{ijk+} (i.e. Table 3.7). The actual latent class model corresponding to (3.10) is

$$\log(m_{hij+}) = \text{CONST} + \text{CIS-R}(h) + \text{GHQ}(i) + \text{HADS}(j)$$
$$+ \log[\Sigma_k \exp{(\text{LC}(k) + \text{CIS-R}(h) \cdot \text{LC}(k)}$$
$$+ \text{GHQ}(i) \cdot \text{LC}(k) + \text{HADS}(j) \cdot \text{LC}(k))] \qquad (3.11)$$

Details of how to fit a model such as this can be found in Agresti (1992) and in Rindskopf (1992). They involve fitting generalised linear models with *composite link functions* (Thompson and Baker, 1981). We do not wish to dwell on the technical details here, however, but simply look at the resulting output. Table 3.8 provides both parameter estimates and fitted values (there are no degrees of freedom to test the fit of the model – it is an exact description of the data when we only have three observed indicators). The parameters corresponding to the two-way interactions are, of course, interpreted as the logarithm of odds-ratios. First, let us look at these parameter estimates. The log(odds-ratios) for the association of the latent class with the CIS-R, the GHQ and

Table 3.8   Results of fitting a latent class model to the CIS-R data

(a) Parameter estimates

Parameter	Estimate	Standard error
CONST	3.549	0.1700
LC	−5.091	0.8741
CISR	−1.969	0.6668
GHQ	−2.843	0.9631
HAD	−2.201	0.5769
LC*CISR	3.740	0.8021
LC*GHQ	4.359	1.0350
LC*HAD	3.982	0.7292

(b) Fitted values

LC	CISR	GHQ	HAD	Count
1	1	1	1	34.78
1	1	1	2	3.85
1	1	2	1	2.03
1	1	2	2	0.22
1	2	1	1	4.85
1	2	1	2	0.54
1	2	2	1	0.28
1	2	2	2	0.03
2	1	1	1	0.21
2	1	1	2	1.27
2	1	2	1	0.97
2	1	2	2	5.78
2	2	1	1	1.26
2	2	1	2	7.46
2	2	2	1	5.73
2	2	2	2	33.99

Table 3.9 Marginal two-way tables obtained from the fitted values in Table 3.8 (rounded to whole numbers for ease of interpretation)

CIS-R by latent class

		CIS-R	
		No	Yes
LC	No	42	5
	Yes	8	48

Sensitivity = 86%

Specificity = 89%

GHQ by latent class

		GHQ	
		No	Yes
LC	No	44	3
	Yes	10	46

Sensitivity = 82%

Specificity = 94%

HADS by latent class

		HADS	
		No	Yes
LC	No	41	6
	Yes	8	48

Sensitivity = 86%

Specificity = 87%

the HADS are 3.740, 4.359 and 3.982, respectively. They are all pretty similar and all very high (a log-odds-ratio of 4 corresponding to an actual odds-ratio of about 55). This is what one would expect in this situation. But what about sensitivity and specificity? These one can calculate from the fitted values in Table 3.8. Table 3.9 provides the required two-way marginal tables of fitted values (indicator by latent class) for each of the three methods of case definition. It also provides the estimates of sensitivity and specificity for each of the three indicators. Typically, sensitivity is about 86% and specificity about 90%.

It is possible to extend this methodology to cope with data from two-phase surveys. In this case we have missing data on two variables. The latent class is, of course, missing for everyone. The interview is missing for those screened but not included in phase two of the survey. The use of composite link functions for this situation is described by Rindskopf (1992), to which the interested reader is referred for further details.

Table 3.10 Alternative parametrisation for a latent class model with three indicators

Indicator 1	Indicator 2	Indicator 3	Expected probability
case	case	case	$\pi\alpha_1\alpha_2\alpha_3 + (1-\pi)\phi_1\phi_2\phi_3$
case	case	non-case	$\pi\alpha_1\alpha_2(1-\alpha_3) + (1-\pi)\phi_1\phi_2(1-\phi_3)$
case	non-case	case	$\pi\alpha_1(1-\alpha_2)\alpha_3 + (1-\pi)\phi_1(1-\phi_2)\phi_3$
case	non-case	non-case	$\pi\alpha_1(1-\alpha_2)(1-\alpha_3) + (1-\pi)\phi_1(1-\phi_2)(1-\phi_3)$
non-case	case	case	$\pi(1-\alpha_1)\alpha_2\alpha_3 + (1-\pi)(1-\phi_1)\phi_2\phi_3$
non-case	case	non-case	$\pi(1-\alpha_1)\alpha_2(1-\alpha_3) + (1-\pi)(1-\phi_1)\phi_2(1-\phi_3)$
non-case	non-case	case	$\pi(1-\alpha_1)(1-\alpha_2)\alpha_3 + (1-\pi)(1-\phi_1)(1-\phi_2)\phi_3$
non-case	non-case	non-case	$\pi(1-\alpha_1)(1-\alpha_2)(1-\alpha_3)$ $+(1-\pi)(1-\phi_1)(1-\phi_2)(1-\phi_3)$

Readers already familiar with latent class models for data to evaluate diagnostic tests, for example, may be used to a completely different approach to parametrisation and model fitting. Returning to the simple cross-sectional survey (i.e. data not collected via double sampling) we could start by first postulating a latent class (illness) with a true but unknown prevalence of π. We also have three conditionally independent indicators of illness with sensitivities of α_1, α_2 and α_3, respectively (α being equivalent to $(1-\delta)$ of Section 3.5). Similarly, let their specificities be $(1-\phi_1)$, $(1-\phi_2)$ and $(1-\phi_3)$. The predicted probabilities for the different combinations of observed results are given in Table 3.10. These *multinomial* probabilities can be fitted to the observed table of counts directly using maximum likelihood methods and the results will be in full agreement with those found using composite link functions. Which approach is preferred is merely a matter of taste and (of course) availability of software (see Dunn, 1989, or Bartholomew, 1987). What consideration of Table 3.10 does do, however, is to prompt us to ask 'What is the best estimate of the prevalence, π?' Returning to the fitted values in Table 3.8, the prevalence defined by LC is 55%. This is only slightly higher than that defined by the CIS-R (52%). We will return to the problems of prevalence estimation using multiple indicators in Chapter 5.

4

Hidden variables and multiple indicators

4.1   Introduction

In this chapter we abandon all pretence of having error-free measuring instruments or gold standards. Knowing that psychiatrists and other clinicians frequently disagree over diagnostic labels or the severity of problems – even after the use of a structured in-depth interview – leads us to conclude that it is preferable explicitly to acknowledge this characteristic of their assessments in our statistical models. We start by treating all assessments, some of which might in the past have been treated as if they were infallible, as alternative, fallible, indicators of the construct which they have been designed to measure. We then evaluate, through the use of appropriate statistical models, the relative merits of these alternative indicators. This evaluation may involve the investigation of both an instrument's reliability and its validity. Much of this chapter is, in fact, concerned with factor analysis models to explain the patterns of covariance (correlation) between the results of administering three or more measuring devices to each member of an appropriate (hopefully large) sample of subjects.

We start our detailed discussion of latent variable models with a model which has its origins in the work of the psychologist Charles Spearman (Spearman, 1904). Spearman was concerned with the measurement of intellectual abilities and postulated that a person's score or examination result for one particular intellectual test or academic discipline is correlated with those from other tests or examinations because of that person's general ability to carry out cognitive tasks (i.e. the person's intelligence). Bright people, on average, are good at all the tasks; those not so bright have difficulty doing any of them. Spearman postulated that a score for a specific task was a linear combination of two components or factors: a *common factor* (intelligence – 'G') common to all tests and a *specific factor* unique to that test under consideration.

Here we consider the measurement of the severity of symptoms of psychological distress as measured by the GHQ, the HADS or the CIS-R (Lewis *et al.*,

1992). We postulate that the three measures have something in common – severity of distress. We also acknowledge that they will also have a component that is specific to each of the three indicators. By explicitly formulating this hypothesis in terms of a statistical model we can study its predictions for the data and hope to learn something about the measures' performance. This is the subject of the next section. Following that we then enrich our model (and the data that we wish to explain) and explore the implications in further detail.

4.2   A single common factor model: the CIS-R data

4.2.1   The measurement model

The following measurement model may be postulated to explain the relationships between the scores from the CIS-R, GHQ and the HADS:

$$\text{CIS-R} = \alpha_c + \beta_c F + E_c$$

$$\text{GHQ} = \alpha_g + \beta_g F + E_g \tag{4.1}$$

$$\text{HADS} = \alpha_h + \beta_h F + E_h$$

where F is a *latent variable* (common factor) representing a subject's psychological stress or severity of illness. The Es are specific factors – those parts of the observed measurements that are specific (i.e. not in common) to each of the indicators. The F and the Es are assumed to be mutually uncorrelated. For the time being the specific factors will be assumed to be simple measurement errors (but see below). A graphical representation of the model (a *path diagram*) is shown in Figure 4.1. In this model, the observed measurements (CIS-R, GHQ and HADS), F and the Es are all random variables. Let the population mean of the Fs be μ_F. Fitting our measurement model to an observed set of data is a simple example of *confirmatory factor analysis* (*CFA*) and the regression coefficients (the βs) relating the common factor, F, to the observed scores are in this context known as *factor loadings*. Assuming that measurement errors are uncorrelated to the true values, then the variance of F, denoted by σ_F^2, together with the variances of the Es, denoted by σ_c^2, σ_g^2 and σ_h^2 for the CIS-R, GHQ and HADS, respectively, jointly predict the variances, covariances and means of the observed scores as in Table 4.1.

For the time being we will ignore μ_F and the αs and concentrate on the estimation of the parameters contributing to the pattern of variances and covariances. Given an observed variance–covariance matrix for a set of three measurements on each of a sample of subjects we can simply equate these summary statistics to their predicted values and solve the resulting six simultaneous equations for the unknown parameters (β_c, β_g, β_h, σ_c^2, σ_g^2, σ_h^2 and σ_F^2). But there is a catch! Note that there are seven parameters describing the pattern of variances and covariances, but only six independent summary statistics from which to estimate them. The model is *under-identified*. The problem arises from the fact that we have not fixed the scale of measurement. As it expands and contracts (via changes in σ_F^2) the βs will adjust accordingly (but note that their values relative to one another will remain the same). So, we need to do something to fix the scale of measurement. One way of doing this (which we

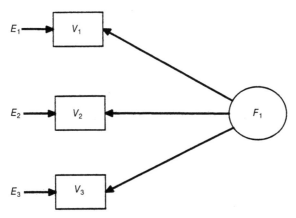

Figure 4.1   Path diagram illustrating Spearman's single common factor model for the CIS-R data.

Key:

Factors are represented within circles

Observed variables are represented within squares

F_1 – the single common factor

V_1 – the Revised Clinical Interview Schedule (CIS-R)

V_2 – the General Health Questionnaire (GHQ)

V_3 – the Hospital Anxiety and Depression Scale (HADS)

E_1, E_2 and E_3 – residuals associated with V_1, V_2 and V_3, respectively

will use here) is to fix the value of σ_F^2 to be 1, on the assumption that the scale of measurement for a psychiatric, behavioural or social indicator is usually completely arbitrary. An alternative would be to set one of the βs (that for the CIS-R, for example) to be 1. Having introduced the constraint on the variance of F the estimation problem is now straightforward. Let the observed (estimated) covariance between the CIS-R and GHQ, for example, be represented by s_{cg}, with the observed variance of the CIS-R being s_{cc}. Then, it is straightforward to show that the remaining six parameters are estimated as

Table 4.1   CIS-R data: expected values for Spearman's single factor model

(a) Covariance matrix

	CIS-R	GHQ	HADS
CIS-R	$\beta_c^2\sigma_F^2 + \sigma_c^2$		
GHQ	$\beta_c\beta_g\sigma_F^2$	$\beta_g^2\sigma_F^2 + \sigma_g^2$	
HADS	$\beta_c\beta_h\sigma_F^2$	$\beta_g\beta_h\sigma_F^2$	$\beta_h^2\sigma_F^2 + \sigma_h^2$

(b) Means

CIS-R	$\mu_c = \alpha_c + \beta_g\mu_F$
GHQ	$\mu_g = \alpha_g + \beta_g\mu_F$
HADS	$\mu_h = \alpha_h + \beta_h\mu_F$

Table 4.2 CIS-R data: estimators for Spearman's common factor model

Parameter	Estimate
β_c	$\sqrt{s_{cg}s_{ch}/s_{gh}}$
β_g	$\sqrt{s_{cg}s_{gh}/s_{ch}}$
β_h	$\sqrt{s_{ch}s_{gh}/s_{cg}}$
σ_c^2	$s_{cc} - s_{cg}s_{ch}/s_{gh}$
σ_g^2	$s_{gg} - s_{cg}s_{gh}/s_{ch}$
σ_h^2	$s_{hh} - s_{ch}s_{gh}/s_{cg}$
$\alpha_c\ (=\mu_c)$	mean(CIS-R)
$\alpha_g\ (=\mu_g)$	mean(GHQ)
$\alpha_h\ (=\mu_h)$	mean(HADS)

in Table 4.2. Similarly, we can equate observed and predicted means to solve for α_c, α_g, α_h and μ_F. Again there is an identifiability problem and we solve this by setting $\mu_F = 0$ (and, again, there are mathematically equivalent alternatives such as setting $\alpha_c = 0$). Having done this, we have estimates provided in Table 4.2.

4.2.2   Reliability and instrument precision

The proportion of variability of a given measure or indicator that is explained by variation in the common factor (or factors in more complex examples involving more than one common factor) is known as the communality of the measure. If the specific factors are just measurement errors then it should be clear from reference to Chapter 2 that the communality of a measure is also equivalent to its reliability. In the above model it follows that

$$R_c = \frac{\beta_c^2}{\beta_c^2 + \sigma_c^2}$$

and, similarly,

$$R_g = \frac{\beta_g^2}{\beta_g^2 + \sigma_g^2} \tag{4.2}$$

$$R_c = \frac{\beta_h^2}{\beta_h^2 + \sigma_h^2}$$

Instrument precision for the CIS-R is given by the reciprocal of the estimate of σ_c^2 (remember that the instrument's standard error of measurement is the square root of this variance). For comparison of instruments, however, we are likely to want to allow for their differing scales of measurement. Here the comparative precision is given by the ratio β_c^2/σ_c^2 (attributed to Frederick Mosteller – see Cochran, 1968).

4.2.3   Working with standardised scores

Suppose that we wish to analyse a correlation matrix rather than the corresponding matrix of variances and covariances. This is equivalent to first standardising the original measures to have zero mean and unit variance. The simplified model is now:

$$\text{CIS-R} = \lambda_c F + e_c$$

$$\text{GHQ} = \lambda_g F + e_g \qquad (4.3)$$

$$\text{HADS} = \lambda_h F + e_h$$

where the λs are standardised regression coefficients (corresponding to the unstandardised βs in the above model). The e's are the rescaled measurement errors (again corresponding to the Es in the above model). The λs are estimated by:

$$\lambda_c = \frac{r_{cg}r_{ch}}{r_{gh}}$$

$$\lambda_g = \frac{r_{cg}r_{gh}}{r_{ch}} \qquad (4.4)$$

$$\lambda_h = \frac{r_{ch}r_{gh}}{r_{cg}}$$

where the r's are the observed product–moment correlations between pairs of variables. Note that the *communalities* (equivalent to reliabilities in the single common factor model) of the CIS-R, the GHQ and the HADS are now simply λ_c^2, λ_g^2 and λ_h^2, respectively and that the variances of the rescaled measurement errors for the CIS-R, GHQ and HADS are $1 - \lambda_c^2$, $1 - \lambda_g^2$ and $1 - \lambda_h^2$, respectively.

4.2.4   A look at the data

Table 4.3 provides the summary statistics required to fit the simple factor analysis model to data on the CIS-R, GHQ and HADS (Lewis *et al.*, 1992). Note that there are two CIS-R scores – the interview was, in fact, carried out twice on each subject – the initial score being CIS-R1 and the retest being CIS-R2. For the time being, however, we will ignore CIS-R2. Before considering factor models, however, we will have a look at the raw data. Figure 4.2 provides scatter plots for each pair of measures. It is clear that the measures are all reasonably highly correlated and there are no obvious signs of outliers or other troublesome observations. One thing is clear, however: the measures are all skewed. There is a concentration of data points in the bottom left of all of the plots. Later in this chapter we will be using fitting methods based on maximum likelihood for data that is assumed to be multivariate normal. Departure from multivariate normality will affect the validity of the standard errors of parameter estimates, confidence intervals for parameters, and also goodness of fit and other significance tests. But departure from normality will have very little impact on the values of the parameter estimates themselves. In the

Table 4.3   Summary statistics for the CIS-R, GHQ and HADS scores (data from the study of Lewis *et al.*, 1992)

Sample size $(N) = 98$

(a) Covariance matrix

	GHQ	HADS	CIS-R1	CIS-R2
GHQ	36.7944			
HADS	32.6451	50.6031		
CIS-R1	43.7913	55.5177	100.139	
CIS-R2	44.3509	55.7599	94.8127	100.976

(b) Correlations

	GHQ	HADS	CIS-R1	CIS-R2
GHQ	1.000			
HADS	0.7566	1.000		
CIS-R1	0.7214	0.7799	1.000	
CIS-R2	0.6941	0.7441	0.8994	1.000

(c) Means

GHQ	HADS	CIS-R1	CIS-R2
12.2245	10.9286	13.6020	12.8163

(d) Standard deviations

GHQ	HADS	CIS-R1	CIS-R2
6.0658	7.1136	10.0070	10.5345

case of fitting a simple common factor model to data from three instruments the parameter estimates given in the above section are **not**, however, dependent on any distributional assumptions.

Returning to Table 4.3, the unstandardised loading for CIS-R1 (β_c) is estimated by $\sqrt{s_{cg}s_{ch}/s_{gh}} = \sqrt{43.7913 \times 55.5177/32.6451} = 8.629$. The corresponding error variance (σ_c^2) is estimated by $100.139 - (43.7913 \times 55.5177/32.6451) = 100.139 - 8.629^2 = 25.674$. The standardised loading (λ_c) is estimated by $\sqrt{r_{cg}r_{ch}/r_{gh}} = 0.862$. The reliability of the CIS-R1 scores is given by $8.629^2/100.139 = 0.744$. Note that, as expected, this is the square of the standardised loading (i.e. 0.862^2). Table 4.4 contains estimates for both the unstandardised and standardised data. These estimates are provided by the software package EQS (Bentler, 1995). The standard errors of these estimates have been calculated via maximum likelihood (assuming multivariate normality) and should, therefore, be treated with caution. The EQS program is listed in full in Appendix 4A.

The striking thing about the results is that there is no evidence at all that the interview (the CIS-R) is performing significantly better than the screening questionnaires (the GHQ and HADS). In fact, the reliability of the HADS appears to be the best of the three. These results should be interpreted with extreme caution, however. We should not fall into the trap of thinking that the common factor is identical to the true but unknown severity score. It is

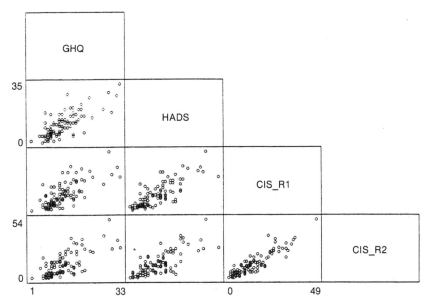

Figure 4.2   A scatter plot matrix for the CIS-R data (data from Lewis *et al.*, 1992).
Key:
GHQ – General Health Questionnaire
HADS – Hospital Anxiety and Depression Scale
CIS_R1 – 1st interview using the Revised Clinical Interview Schedule
CIS_R2 – 2nd interview using the Revised Clinical Interview Schedule

Table 4.4   Results of fitting a single factor model to GHQ, HADS and CIS-R1 scores

(a) Unstandardised estimates

Parameter	Estimate	Standard error
β_c	8.629	0.843
β_g	5.074	0.518
β_h	6.434	0.585
σ_c^2	25.674	5.647
σ_g^2	11.044	2.169
σ_h^2	9.212	2.721

(b) Standardised solution

Parameter	Estimate	Reliability
λ_c	0.862	$\lambda_c^2 = 0.743$
λ_g	0.837	$\lambda_g^2 = 0.817$
λ_h	0.904	$\lambda_h^2 = 0.701$

merely a consensus. If there is a source of variation (other than severity itself) that is common to the two screening questionnaires then this will tend to be incorporated into this consensus, thus making the CIS-R appear to be performing less well than one might have expected. This will be discussed in further detail in the following section.

4.3　Model-fitting and inference

In the above section we have fitted a model by simply equating an observed covariance matrix with one predicted by our model parameters and then solving to obtain our estimates of the parameters. Typically, however, we will find parameter estimates by using iterative numerical methods to minimise the difference between the two matrices. In general, if we represent an observed covariance matrix by S (with elements $\{s_{ij}\}$) and the covariance matrix predicted by the parameter estimates by Σ (with elements $\{\sigma_{ij}\}$) then the residual covariance is the difference $S - \Sigma$. The elements of this residual matrix are simply $\{s_{ij} - \sigma_{ij}\}$. (On the assumption that the context will make it clear whether we are discussing the parameter itself or its estimate, we do not bother with the customary 'hat' to indicate that we are referring to an estimate.) If the parameters of any given model are represented by the vector $\theta^T = (\theta_1, \theta_2, \ldots, \theta_t)$, where t is the number of parameters to be estimated, then we can be more explicit in our description of a particular predicted covariance matrix by using the term $\Sigma(\theta)$. The most commonly used fitting criterion involves minimising

$$F_{\mathrm{ML}} = \mathrm{tr}(S\Sigma^{-1}) + \log|\Sigma| - \log|S| - q \qquad (4.5)$$

where q is the number of latent variables or factors. The symbol 'tr' is the trace operator indicating the sum of the diagonal elements of a matrix. F_{ML} produces estimates that are maximum likelihood, **provided that the data are multivariate normal**. Other fitting criteria are discussed in Bollen (1989).

It clearly makes sense to use the optimal value of the fitting criterion, such as the minimum value of F_{ML}, as a measure of the goodness of fit of the model: the lower the value the better the fit. In fact, assuming multivariate normality, it is possible to show that F_{ML} has (for sufficiently large sample sizes) a chi-squared distribution under the null hypothesis that the covariance matrix is of the form predicted by the model. The degrees of freedom for the chi-squared distribution (ν) is given by

$$\nu = \tfrac{1}{2}p(p+1) - t \qquad (4.6)$$

where p is the number of measured variables and t the number of estimated (free) parameter values.

Having fitted a particular model, the elements of the residual matrix, $\{s_{ij} - \sigma_{ij}\}$, should be relatively small and evenly spread among the variables if the model is a reasonable one for the data. Large residuals associated with specific variables are an indication of poor fit. The output provided by computer software usually also includes summaries of standardised residuals of the form $\{r_{ij} - \sigma_{ij}/\sqrt{s_{ii}s_{jj}}\}$, where r_{ij} is the observed correlation between variables i and j.

The standardised residuals (based on correlations) are easier to interpret than unstandardised ones (based on covariances) since they are not dependent on the scale of the observed measurements.

If we have measurements that are clearly not normally distributed then we have to be cautious about the interpretation of goodness of fit (chi-squared) statistics and the standard errors of the parameter estimates. One possibility is to transform the data to normality (or at least symmetry) but this is not always possible, particularly with data such as severity measures, which often have a modal value at zero. Another possibility is to estimate the parameters of the model using the inappropriate maximum likelihood criterion, but then to obtain estimates of the standard errors by a method robust to this incorrect model specification. Jackknife and bootstrap are two possibilities (see Dunn, 1989). A more easily implemented approach is to use a 'sandwich' parameter covariance estimator such as that of White (1982), Huber (1967), Browne and Shapiro (1988) or Satorra and Bentler (1990). In this text we will provide robust chi-squared statistics and robust standard errors for the parameters of factor analysis and other covariance components models (via EQS) using the method of Satorra and Bentler.

4.4   Another look at the CIS-R data

This time we start by fitting a single common factor model to all four scores: the GHQ, HADS and both CIS-R measures. We introduce a couple of *a priori* constraints, however, to make the two CIS-R measures parallel (equal loadings and equal error variances). The EQS program is given in Appendix 4B. The model is *over-identified* (basically, there are fewer parameters to be estimated than there are independent elements in the covariance matrix) and so we use maximum likelihood to fit the model to the data. The results are given in Table 4.5. The estimated reliabilities for the CIS-R, GHQ and HADS are 0.889, 0.591 and 0.674. At least these appear to be in the expected rank order. But, the goodness of fit chi-square is 17.659 with four degrees of freedom ($P = 0.001$). The robust chi-square is 12.187 ($P = 0.016$). The model does not fit at all well. Examination of the standardised residuals yields absolute values in the range 0.008–0.054 for all of the correlations except that between the GHQ and HADS ($+0.125$) – i.e. this correlation is higher than that predicted by the model. Note that the robust standard errors are consistently higher than those provided via maximum likelihood.

One obvious solution is to acknowledge that the errors in the two CIS-R scores are likely to be correlated. This could arise from memory effects or from the fact that there is something common to the two CIS-R measures that is not common to either the GHQ or the HADS. If we introduce the required correlation then the resulting chi-square drops to 3.279 with three degrees of freedom (the corresponding robust chi-square is 2.906). The model now fits well. The standardised estimates are given in Table 4.6(a). But what if we allow correlated errors for the GHQ and HADS instead? The model is exactly equivalent to the one in which correlated errors for the two CIS-R scores are allowed. The goodness of fit statistics are identical. There is no way in which we can distinguish the two models. The parameter estimates change,

Table 4.5 Results of fitting a single factor model to GHQ, HADS, CIS-R1 and CIS-R2 scores

(a) Unstandardised estimates

Parameter	Estimate	Standard error (s.e.)	Robust s.e.
β_c	9.694	0.740	0.913
β_g	4.664	0.526	0.665
β_h	5.843	0.597	0.653
σ_c^2	11.593	1.650	2.051
σ_g^2	15.037	2.335	2.639
σ_h^2	16.463	2.654	3.093

(b) Standardised solution

Parameter	Estimate	Reliability
λ_c	0.943	$\lambda_c^2 = 0.889$
λ_g	0.769	$\lambda_g^2 = 0.591$
λ_h	0.821	$\lambda_h^2 = 0.674$

however. These are given in Table 4.6(b). Note the impact that the changing model specification has on the reliabilities of the three measures.

Two further ways of specifying the well-fitting model involve the introduction of method-specific factors: one can introduce a method-specific factor for the two CIS-R scores or, alternatively, a similar factor can be introduced for the two questionnaires. One such model for the standardised scores, for example, is

$$\text{CIS-R1} = \lambda_c F_1 + \lambda_{cs} F_2 + e_c$$
$$\text{CIS-R2} = \lambda_c F_1 + \lambda_{cs} F_2 + e_c$$
$$\text{GHQ} = \lambda_g F_1 + e_g \tag{4.7}$$
$$\text{HADS} = \lambda_h F_1 + e_h$$

where F_1 is the factor common to all four measures and F_2 is a factor specific to the CIS-R. Again the CIS-R scores are constrained to be parallel and the variances of the two factors are fixed at 1. Again, it makes no difference to the goodness of fit and, indeed, the models are both equivalent to those in which correlated errors are specified – see Table 4.6(c) and 4.6(d) for the standardised estimates. The four sub-tables in Table 4.6 should, we hope, give the reader some insight into what is going on. The key thing to remember is that for any given covariance matrix there is unlikely to be a unique correct model. And quite often the interpretation is dependent on the specification chosen. Clearly in this example the reliability of the measures is dependent on the model chosen (depending whether the specific components are regarded as a stable component of a given score, or whether they are to be regarded as correlated measurement errors). And what about validity? That, too, is dependent on model specification. To resolve these problems, however, we need a

Table 4.6   Alternative models for CIS-R data (standardised solutions)

Model (a) – correlated errors for CIS-R1 and CIS-R2

Parameter	Estimate	Reliability
λ_c	0.844	$\lambda_c^2 = 0.712$
λ_g	0.838	$\lambda_g^2 = 0.702$
λ_h	0.902	$\lambda_h^2 = 0.814$

Model (b) – correlated errors for GHQ and HAD

Parameter	Estimate	Reliability
λ_c	0.948	$\lambda_c^2 = 0.899$
λ_g	0.746	$\lambda_g^2 = 0.557$
λ_h	0.803	$\lambda_h^2 = 0.645$

Model (c) – specific factor for CIS-R1 and CIS-R2

Parameter	Estimate	Parameter	Estimate	Reliability
λ_c	0.844	λ_{cs}	0.432	$\lambda_c^2 + \lambda_{cs}^2 = 0.899$
λ_g	0.838			$\lambda_g^2 = 0.702$
λ_h	0.902			$\lambda_h^2 = 0.814$

Model (d) – specific factor for GHQ and HAD

Parameter	Estimate	Parameter	Estimate	Reliability
λ_c	0.948			$\lambda_c^2 = 0.899$
λ_g	0.746	λ_{gs}	0.429	$\lambda_g^2 + \lambda_{gs}^2 = 0.741$
λ_h	0.803	λ_{hs}	0.366	$\lambda_h^2 + \lambda_{hs}^2 = 0.779$

richer data set – see Section 4.6. First we consider simple models with two common factors.

4.5   Two-factor models

Let us have another look at the GHQ data in Table 2.1 and think how we might explore the covariance or correlation matrix for the four GHQ scores (Odd1, Even1, Odd2 and Even2) in terms of a factor analysis model. Table 4.7 provides us with the required summary statistics for these data. Here we will regard the sum of the odd items and the sum of the even items to be alternative forms of the test. We assume that there has been some temporal change in the true levels of distress between test and retest. Let Odd1 and Even1 be parallel tests, each being a manifest indicator for a factor, F_1. Similarly, let Odd2 and Even2 also be parallel tests, but each of these an indicator of a separate factor, F_2. We

Table 4.7 Summary statistics for the GHQ data in Table 2.1 (data from Dunn, 1992)

Sample size $(N) = 12$

(a) Correlations

	Odd1	Even1	Odd2	Even2
Odd1	1.0000			
Even1	0.8645	1.0000		
Odd2	0.9008	0.7516	1.0000	
Even2	0.8597	0.8682	0.9075	1.0000

(b) Standard deviations

	Odd1	Even1	Odd2	Even2
	3.5792	3.0189	3.0451	3.1909

expect F_1 and F_2 to be highly correlated, with the possibility that they might be replaced by a single common factor, F. The measurement model has the following structure:

$$\text{Odd1} = \beta_e F_1 + E_1$$

$$\text{Even1} = \beta_e F_1 + E_2$$

$$\text{Odd2} = \beta_e F_2 + E_3$$ (4.8)

$$\text{Even2} = \beta_e F_2 + E_4$$

Note that the value of β_e has been assumed to be the same for all four indicators. Let us also assume that $\text{Var}(E_1) = \text{Var}(E_3) = \text{Var}(E_2) = \text{Var}(E_4) = \sigma_e^2$. Let the variances of F_1 and of F_2 both be 1. The model is illustrated in Figure 4.3. What are the predicted variances and covariances? It follows from the usual independence assumptions that the expected covariance matrix has the structure given in Table 4.8, where ρ is the correlation between F_1 and F_2.

Note that if we were to equate observed and expected covariances/variances and solve the resulting simultaneous equations then there would be several possible solutions for the model's parameters (that is, the model is overidentified). Again, we need to use maximum likelihood to find the best parameter estimates. In this example the GHQ scores are approximately multivariate normal. Appendix 4C gives the EQS program listing for this model.

The resulting chi-square to test goodness of fit is 10.906 based on seven degrees of freedom ($P = 0.143$). The fit is reasonable. The estimate of ρ is 0.961. The reliability of the observed scores is $0.927^2 = 0.859$. The obvious question is 'is the correlation ρ significantly different from 1?' That is, are F_1 and F_2 the same? Fitting a single factor model to these data (with all other parameters constrained as before) produces a chi-square of 11.655 based on eight degrees of freedom ($P = 0.167$). The difference in chi-squares provides a test of significance of $\rho = 1$ against the alternative $\rho < 1$. It is 0.749 with one degree of freedom (clearly not significant). The revised estimate of the reliabilities for the observed sub-scales is $0.925^2 = 0.856$.

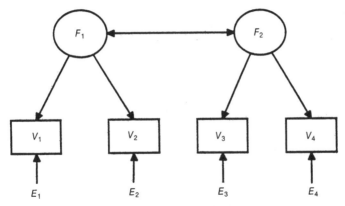

Figure 4.3   Path diagram for a two-factor model of GHQ scores.
Key:
F_1 – psychological distress at time 1
F_2 – psychological distress at time 2
V_1 – Odd1 (sum of odd items at time 1)
V_2 – Even1 (sum of even items at time 1)
V_3 – Odd2 (sum of odd items at time 2)
V_4 – Even2 (sum of even items at time 2)
E_1 to E_4, disturbance terms associated with V_1 to V_4, respectively
Note: The double-headed arrow linking F_1 and F_2 indicates correlation, without an implied direction of influence or causality.

One final point: these reliabilities are equivalent to those obtained from a mixed model ANOVA – see Chapter 2 – with fixed effects for time (i.e. they are product–moment correlations). If we were interested in intraclass correlations then we would have to fit models incorporating means as well as variances and covariances in our model. The mean of Odd1 and Odd2, for example, would have to be constrained to be equal, as would that of Even1 and Even2. This is quite straightforward but is beyond the scope of this text. The joint modelling of means and covariances in EQS is described in detail in Dunn, Everitt and Pickles (1993) and briefly in Chapter 7 of the present text.

Another approach to the modelling of these data could have involved a single common factor together with a method factor associated either with the odd sub-scores or the even ones (but not both, because of problems of identifiability). This would be analogous to the models used for fitting the CIS-R

Table 4.8   Expected covariance matrix for the two-factor model describing the GHQ data*

	Odd1	Even1	Odd2	Even2
Odd1	$\beta_e^2 + \sigma_e^2$			
Even1	β_e^2	$\beta_e^2 + \sigma_e^2$		
Odd2	$\rho\beta_e^2$	$\rho\beta_e^2$	$\beta_e^2 + \sigma_e^2$	
Even2	$\rho\beta_e^2$	$\rho\beta_e^2$	β_e^2	$\beta_e^2 + \sigma_e^2$

* ρ is the correlation between F_1 and F_2.

data in Section 4.4. In both cases we are attempting to measure a single trait through the use of two or more independent methods. We will not discuss this question in any further detail here, but will move on to the more general problem of jointly assessing two or more distinct traits through the use of two or more methods.

4.6   Multitrait–multimethod (MTMM) models

In Chapter 2 we were primarily concerned with reliability estimation, while in Chapter 3 the main area of interest was in validity. In the present chapter we have been tempted to blur the distinctions between the two, but we have mainly been concerned with reliability and precision. Here we will try to draw the different strands together. In a very influential paper, Campbell and Fiske (1959) produced the following statement:

> Reliability is the agreement between two efforts to measure the same trait through maximally similar methods. Validity is represented in the agreement between two methods to measure the same trait through maximally different methods.

They went on to suggest that reliability and validity should be jointly assessed through the use of a *multitrait–multimethod* (*MTMM*) approach. Here two or more traits in a sample of participants is assessed using two or more measurement techniques. In child psychiatry, for example, one might be interested in measuring hyperactivity and the extent of conduct disorder using information provided by multiple informants (peer, teacher or parent, for example). The consistency of the teachers' reports gives one a handle on reliability; the correlation or association between the views of teachers and parents tells us about validity. Note that we have abandoned all reference to gold standards or to any idea that one of the methods of assessment might be free from error.

Table 4.9(a) is an example of a correlation matrix derived from the results of a multitrait–multimethod study of childhood anxiety and depression (Cole *et al.*, 1997). Table 4.9(b) is the correlation matrix from a similar study of childhood depression and aggression (Messer and Gross, 1994). The correlations from Cole *et al.* are those obtained after deleting overlapping items from the assessment rating scales. The striking thing about these two matrices is their similarity. Almost equally striking is the fact that the within-method, cross-trait correlations (those in bold) are relatively high compared with the cross-method, within-trait correlations (those underlined). High cross-method, within-trait correlations are evidence of what Campbell and Fiske call *convergent validity*: the agreement of different methods in measuring the same trait. Low correlations elsewhere (both within-method, cross-trait and cross-method, cross-trait) are indicative of *discriminant validity*. Of course, both convergent and discriminant validity are aspects of the assessment methods' *construct validity*. Neither of these two correlation matrices is displaying either high convergent validity or high discriminant validity. The method of assessment appears to be dominating the results, irrespective of what trait is being assessed.

To get a bit more enlightenment we will fit a confirmatory factor analysis model to the Cole *et al.* correlations. Quoting Cole *et al.* (1997):

Table 4.9 Examples of multitrait–multimethod correlation matrices

(a) Childhood depression and anxiety (from Cole *et al.*, 1997)

	V_1	V_2	V_3	V_4	V_5	V_6	V_7	V_8
Depression								
V_1 – Self	1.00							
V_2 – Peers	0.21	1.00						
V_3 – Teacher	0.19	0.32	1.00					
V_4 – Parent	0.21	0.32	0.27	1.00				
Anxiety								
V_5 – Self	**0.66**	0.17	0.10	0.16	1.00			
V_6 – Peers	0.18	**0.72**	0.26	0.22	0.10	1.00		
V_7 – Teacher	0.15	0.25	**0.76**	0.25	0.06	0.27	1.00	
V_8 – Parent	0.24	0.33	0.22	**0.72**	0.22	0.25	0.20	1.00
$N = 280$								
Mean	5.98	0.45	17.36	4.23	15.31	0.53	16.37	10.62
S.D.	7.21	0.43	6.02	4.56	9.44	0.39	5.51	6.24

(b) Childhood depression and aggression (from Messer and Gross, 1994)

	V_1	V_2	V_3	V_4	V_5	V_6
Depression						
V_1 – Self	1.00					
V_2 – Peers	0.24	1.00				
V_3 – Teacher	0.19	0.25	1.00			
Aggression						
V_4 – Self	**0.47**	0.13	0.07	1.00		
V_5 – Peers	0.11	**0.49**	0.16	0.24	1.00	
V_6 – Teacher	0.16	0.33	**0.47**	0.28	0.59	1.00
$N = 356$						

Key:
Cross-method, within-trait correlations are underlined.
Within-method, cross-trait correlations are **bold**.

We allowed each measure to load onto exactly two factors, one trait factor and one method factor. For example, we allowed the depression self-report measure to load onto a depression factor and a self-report factor. We fixed all of the other loadings for this measure to be zero. Comparable loadings were allowed (and disallowed) for all of the other measures. Hence we extracted six factors in all: two trait factors (depression symptoms and anxiety symptoms) and four method factors (self-report, peer nomination, teacher rating, and parent report). We allowed the two trait factors to correlate with one another but not with the method factors. Likewise, we allowed the method factors to correlate with one another but not with the trait factors. The only additional assumption built into the model was that the loadings of measures onto the same method factor were constrained to be equal. (Trait factor loadings were not constrained.)

Cole *et al.* comment that the assumption of equal method factor loadings was necessary for the structural identification of the model. Problems of identification – including out-of-range estimates and convergence difficulties – are an important issue in the analysis of MTMM matrices (and many others!) and the interested reader is referred to Kenny and Kashy (1992) for a thorough discussion of these issues.

Cole *et al.*'s model fits the data quite well – the authors reporting a chi-square statistic of 8.45 (with nine degrees of freedom). Repeating their analysis using the summary statistics in Table 4.9(a) produced a chi-square of 7.94 – the difference presumably arising from the fact that the present analysis was based on published summary statistics given to only two decimal places. The present analysis yielded an estimate of the correlation between the two traits of 0.811, and estimates of the correlations between methods ranging from 0.158 to 0.339. We now introduce one further set of constraints: the correlations between method factors are **all** zero. The EQS program for fitting this model is given in Appendix 4D. The resulting chi-square is 15.432 based on 15 degrees of freedom. The difference between the two chi-squares (15.432 – 7.94) is 7.492 with six degrees of freedom – clearly not statistically significant. The estimates of the standardised loadings are provided in Table 4.10. Note (in case of confusion) that, although the unstandardised loadings for the method factors are constrained to be equal across the two traits, this is not the case for the standardised values.

One further model tests whether depression and anxiety might be regarded as a unitary trait. We replace the two trait factors by a single trait factor (equivalent to constraining the correlation between the two factors to be 1) and refit the model. The resulting chi-square is 16.852 with 16 degrees of freedom. Clearly the evidence that anxiety and depression can be measured separately in these children is very weak. The data in Table 4.9(a) refer to third-graders. Cole *et al.* also analysed data from sixth-grade students and in this case the correlation between the two trait factors was lower (about 0.7) and significantly different from 1.

Returning to Table 4.10, we can infer that although each of the assessment methods is likely to be reasonably consistent (reliable) – as indicated by the

Table 4.10   Parameter estimates from CFA of depression/ anxiety correlations (data from Cole *et al.*, 1997)

Two common trait factors, four method factors (standardised results)

$$V_1 = 0.374F_1 + 0.854F_3 + 0.362E_1$$
$$V_2 = 0.617F_1 + 0.623F_4 + 0.481E_2$$
$$V_3 = 0.501F_1 + 0.713F_5 + 0.491E_3$$
$$V_4 = 0.530F_1 + 0.780F_6 + 0.333E_4$$

$$V_5 = 0.279F_2 + 0.652F_3 + 0.705E_5$$
$$V_6 = 0.494F_2 + 0.687F_4 + 0.533E_6$$
$$V_7 = 0.430F_2 + 0.778F_5 + 0.458E_7$$
$$V_8 = 0.540F_2 + 0.570F_6 + 0.620E_8$$

$$\text{Corr}(F_1, F_2) = 0.962$$

sums of the squares of the standardised loadings for the appropriate trait and method loadings – the validities of the measures are all quite poor. The squares of the standardised trait loadings are all pretty low compared to those of the method loadings and, of course, we have the problem of the near-perfect correlation between the trait factors for depression and anxiety.

4.7 Causal indicators

Throughout this chapter, until now, we have explicitly assumed a measurement model or models in which we postulate the existence of a latent variable or variables that in some way 'cause' or lead to the measured indicators. These latent variables 'explain' the covariances or correlations between the observed indicators of a given concept. In the context of an illustrative path diagram, the arrows are directed from the latent variable towards the observed indicator. The latent variable or factor called 'general intelligence', for example, explains a child's ability to carry out a wide variety of cognitive tasks; the ability of a child to carry out a particular mathematical test does not affect his or her intelligence but, instead, is a reflection or manifestation of that intelligence. A factor called 'severity of depression' explains the presence of a range of depressive symptoms. Symptoms are considered to be the effects of the underlying severity of depression and, for this reason, are frequently referred to as *effect indicators* or *indicator variables*. But often it might be much more convincing to think of the so-called causal arrows pointing in the opposite direction: from the observed indicator towards the latent variable. The underlying factor is predicted or influenced by the observed characteristics, states or events.

Consider the measurement of social stress, for example. Stressful life events such as the death of a parent or a spouse, the break-up of a marriage, being a victim of a serious traffic accident or being mugged in the street, lead to severe stress. The life events are clearly the causes of stress rather than the effects of it. The manifest indicators (life events) are the predictors or causes of the postulated concept or latent variable(s) which we choose to call stress: they are *causal indicators* or *causal variables* (Bollen and Lennox, 1991). Fayers *et al.* (1997) discuss causal indicators in the context of the measurement of quality of life (QoL). They argue that QoL questionnaires contain two different types of items. Some of them, such as indicators of symptoms of disease, are causal indicators. The occurrence of these symptoms can cause a change in QoL. A severe state of even a single symptom (such as nausea resulting from chemotherapy for cancer) can lower QoL, although poor QoL does not necessarily imply that a patient suffers from any particular symptom. The same would apply in the case of disabilities, financial hardship or relationship problems. Other questionnaire items indicating, for example, levels of anxiety and depression may, however, be better treated as if they were effect indicators. Here lower QoL leads to more anxiety and depression. Note that it is not always obvious whether a given indicator should be a cause or an effect of a given concept – and there is always the possibility that it serves both functions simultaneously – but Fayers *et al.* (1997) develop some formal quantitative methods to help distinguish them.

What are the consequences of adopting a measurement model involving causal indicators? The first and most obvious one is that the model does not have anything to say about correlations or associations between the indicators. They could be positively correlated (if the result of a particular form of treatment, for example), negatively correlated (if the presence of one indicator tended to be inconsistent with that of another) or have no correlation at all. It would therefore be a nonsense to select items on the basis of their correlation with other items (the idea of having a high internal consistency as measured by Cronbach's alpha coefficient, for example, is of no value here). Leading on from this are the implications for item selection. One usually thinks of the sampling of indicator items or facets of a construct in order to measure it. We select those items which in some way are the best indicators in the sense of having maximal correlation with the construct in question – the selected items being representative of what might have been chosen. We can assess the effects of adding or removing items from a questionnaire in terms of its reliability or internal consistency. Causal indicators, however, operate differently (Bollen and Lennox, 1991). With causal indicators the concept being measured is composed of the effects of all the measured indicators. Omitting one or more of them changes the nature of the concept being measured. With causal indicators we need a census of indicators, not a sample (Bollen and Lennox, 1991).

The idea of causal indicators was first developed by Blalock (1964, 1982) and its implication for the measurement of social constructs has been discussed in detail by Bollen (1984, 1989) and Bollen and Lennox (1991). More recently, Fayers and Hand (1997) and Fayers *et al.* (1997) have carried out a detailed evaluation of the role of causal indicators in the particular context of the measurement of quality of life. In terms of statistical modelling, MacCallum and Browne (1993) have pointed out many of the practical implications (difficulties!) of their use – we will not pursue the matter here.

4.8   Appendix 4

A   EQS program to fit a single factor model to the CIS-R data

```
/TITLE
 Single Factor Model
 CIS-R data (Lewis et al, 1992)
 /SPECIFICATION
 CASES=98;
 VARIABLES=4;
 METHOD=ML;
 MATRIX=CORRELATION;
 ANALYSIS=COVARIANCE;
/LABELS
 V1=GHQ;
 V2=HAD;
 V3=CIS1;
 V4=CIS2;
 F1=SEVERITY;
/EQUATIONS
 V1=1*F1+E1;
```

```
 V2=1*F1+E2;
 V3=1*F1+E3;
 V4=1*F1+E4;
/VARIANCES
 F1=1.0;
 E1 TO E4=3*;
/MATRIX
 1.000
 0.7566 1.000
 0.7214 0.7799 1.000
 0.6941 0.7441 0.8994 1.000
/STANDARD DEVIATIONS
 6.0658 7.1136 10.0070 10.5345
/END
```

B   EQS program to fit a model with a method-specific factor to the CIS-R data

```
/TITLE
 Method-specific factor Model
 CIS-R data (Lewis et al, 1992)
 /SPECIFICATION
 CASES=98;
 VARIABLES=4;
 METHOD=ML;
 MATRIX=CORRELATION;
 ANALYSIS=COVARIANCE;
/LABELS
 V1=GHQ;
 V2=HAD;
 V3=CIS1;
 V4=CIS2;
 F1=SEVERITY;
 F2=CIS-SPECIFIC ERROR;
/EQUATIONS
 V1=1*F1+E1;
 V2=1*F1+E2;
 V3=1*F1+F2+E3;
 V4=1*F1+F2+E4;
/VARIANCES
 F1=1.0; F2=0.1*;
 E1 TO E4=3*;
/MATRIX
 1.000
 0.7566 1.000
 0.7214 0.7799 1.000
 0.6941 0.7441 0.8994 1.000
/STANDARD DEVIATIONS
 6.0658 7.1136 10.0070 10.5345
/END
```

C   EQS program to fit a two-factor model to GHQ data

```
/TITLE
 Two Factor Model
 Data are GHQ scores from 12 students
 Odd vs Even subtotals on two occasions
/SPECIFICATION
 CASES=12;
 VARIABLES=4;
 METHOD=ML;
 MATRIX=CORRELATION;
 ANALYSIS=COVARIANCE;
/LABELS
 V1=ODD1;
 V2=EVEN1;
 V3=ODD2;
 V4=EVEN2;
 F1=DISTRESS1;
 F2=DISTRESS2;
/EQUATIONS
 V1=1*F1+E1;
 V2=1*F1+E2;
 V3=1*F2+E3;
 V4=1*F2+E4;
/VARIANCES
 F1 TO F2=1;
 E1 TO E4=1*;
/COVARIANCES
 F1,F2=0.96*;
/CONSTRAINTS
 (V1,F1)=(V2,F1)=(V3,F2)=(V4,F2);
 (E1,E1)=(E2,E2)=(E3,E3)=(E4,E4);
/MATRIX
 1.000
 0.8645 1.000
 0.9008 0.7516 1.000
 0.8597 0.8682 0.9075 1.000
/STANDARD DEVIATIONS
 3.5792 3.0189 3.0451 3.1909
/END
```

D   EQS program to fit a multitrait–multimethod model for depression and anxiety

```
/TITLE
 Multitrait-multimethod analyses
 Depression & Anxiety data - Cole et al (1997)
 MODIFIED SCALES
/SPECIFICATION
```

```
 CASES=280;
 VARIABLES=8;
 METHOD=ML;
 MATRIX=CORRELATION;
 ANALYSIS=COVARIANCE;
/LABELS
 V1=D-SELF; V2=D-PEER; V3=D-TEACH; V4=D-PARENT;
 V5=A-SELF; V6=A-PEER; V7=A-TEACH; V8=A-PARENT;
 F1=DEPRESSION;
 F2=ANXIETY;
 F3=SELF;
 F4=PEER;
 F5=TEACH;
 F6=PARENT;
/EQUATIONS
 V1=1.3*F1+6.5*F3+E1;
 V2=0.3*F1+0.3*F4+E2;
 V3=1.3*F1+5.0*F5+E3;
 V4=1.5*F1+4.1*F6+E4;
 V5=2.2*F2+6.5*F3+E5;
 V6=0.1*F2+0.3*F4+E6;
 V7=0.3*F2+5.0*F5+E7;
 V8=3.1*F2+4.1*F6+E8;
/VARIANCES
 F1 TO F2=1.0;
 F3 TO F6=1.0;
 E1 TO E8=3*;
/COVARIANCES
 F1,F2=0.81*;
/CONSTRAINTS
 (V1,F3)=(V5,F3);
 (V2,F4)=(V6,F4);
 (V3,F5)=(V7,F5);
 (V4,F6)=(V8,F6);
/MATRIX
 1.00
 0.21 1.00
 0.19 0.32 1.00
 0.21 0.32 0.27 1.00
 0.66 0.17 0.10 0.16 1.00
 0.18 0.72 0.26 0.22 0.10 1.00
 0.15 0.25 0.76 0.25 0.06 0.27 1.00
 0.24 0.33 0.22 0.72 0.22 0.25 0.20 1.00
/STANDARD DEVIATIONS
 7.21 0.43 6.02 4.56 9.44 0.39 5.51 6.24
/END
```

5

Prevalence estimation

5.1   Introduction: survey sampling designs

Suppose that we wish to estimate the prevalence of depression in a small town of, say, ten thousand adult inhabitants. These ten thousand people are our *target population*. Now also suppose that we have a list containing the names of these ten thousand people (the *sampling frame*). Using this list, we wish to draw a representative sample from this population, assess whether each of the selected participants shows evidence of suffering from depression and, finally, use this information to estimate the prevalence of depression in the town. If we choose to assess all ten thousand inhabitants of the town then this would be a complete *census*. A census is rarely feasible, however, and we are usually faced with the problem of how best to draw samples from the sampling frame. The first thing to specify is the size of the sample or, alternatively, the *sampling fraction*, which is the proportion of the total number of subjects to be selected. In order to avoid possible selection biases and to provide us with a valid model for statistical inference, we usually aim to use some sort of *random sampling* mechanism.

Random sampling implies that a participant finishing up in the sample is determined by chance; there is no way of predicting which particular participants will be in the sample. A familiar example is dealing a hand of playing cards. The dealer should have thoroughly shuffled the pack, without being able to see the identity of any of the cards, prior to dealing. The card player receives, for example, a sample of five of the possible 52 cards and the identity of the five cards is completely determined by chance. Dealing a hand of playing cards is, in fact, an example of a particular type of random sampling mechanism: *simple random sampling*. The word 'simple' implies that we can enumerate all the possible samples of a given size which might be drawn and that the probability of obtaining any one of them is equal to that of any other (i.e. the probabilities are all equal). With a pack of 52 there are 2 598 960 different possible hands of five cards. The probability of obtaining any one of them is therefore 1 in 2 598 960. Instead of a simple random sample we might choose to select a *systematic sample* or, alternatively, a *Bernoulli sample*. In a systematic sample we might, for example, select one of the first ten names from the population list (frame) and then systematically select every tenth person until we get to the bottom of the list. Note that, although each person has the same probability of selection, this does not apply to the samples themselves (in the above example samples containing both subject nine and subject ten are impossible). In Bernoulli sampling we consider each possible participant in turn and use a random device to decide whether he or she should be selected – keeping the probability of selection constant for all members of the frame. We could throw a die, for example, and select the person under consideration if we happen to throw a six. Note that in Bernoulli sampling the sample size is not fixed but is a random variable that is distributed according to the familiar *binomial distribution*.

A corollary of the last point is that the sampling fraction is also a random variable rather than a constant that is specified by the design. The ideal approach is usually to aim to use a simple random sample. Systematic sampling is much easier to implement but statistical inference based on systematic sampling is much more problematic (Särndal *et al.*, 1992). Bernoulli sampling is useful when one does not have prior access to a sampling frame (as is systematic sampling for that matter). Here we might, for example, be sampling patients visiting a primary-care clinic on a given day. We might have access to a list of appointees (the sampling frame) but if they have not necessarily made a prior appointment then we will not. One possible approach is to interview (say) every fifth patient entering the clinic (this is systematic sampling as long as we choose the starting point at random). The other possibility is to decide at random whether to interview each patient as he or she arrives, using a fixed selection probability of 1/5 for all patients (Bernoulli sampling).

What other forms of random sampling might be used? Perhaps the most common is a *stratified random sample*. Here we divide our target population into distinct groups or strata. These could be men and women, different age bands, social classes and so on. Having chosen our strata we then proceed to select a simple random sample (but possibly systematic or Bernoulli sample) from each of them. The proportion of subjects sampled from each strata (the sampling fraction) might be constant across all the samples (ensuring that the overall sample has the same composition as the original population) or we might decide that one or more strata might have a higher representation. We may be particularly interested in investigating a relatively rare group for example (those aged over 90 years, say), and comparing them with a similar sized sample from a more common stratum (the middle-aged). Another commonly used sampling mechanism is *cluster sampling*. We might, for example, take a sample of clinics and investigate all patients attending or registered with each of the sampled clinics. A development of this approach is *two-stage sampling*: first we select a sample of clusters (clinics, for example) and then we select a sample of subjects (patients) from within each of the clusters.

Returning to our problem of assessing the prevalence of depression, diagnostic interviews carried out by a clinician are often too expensive and time-consuming to justify their use in the general population where the great majority will not show any signs of psychopathology. However, these problems can often be overcome by making use of a survey design that involves the use of an initial screening test such as a questionnaire, which is inexpensive and relatively easy to use in the field, but thought to be less accurate than use of the formal interview. In order to validate the screening questionnaire a sub-sample of the screened participants can be drawn for comparison with the results of an interview. The latter sub-sample is usually obtained through the use of a *two-phase* or *double sampling* design, with the probability of selection at the second phase being dependent on the results of screening and perhaps other information collected at the first phase. In psychiatry (and in other areas of medical research) the term *two-stage* design is widely used for two-phase or double sampling. This can lead to confusion since two-stage sampling is an already long-established name in survey research for a form of cluster sampling (see previous paragraph and also Cochran, 1977). A two-phase sampling procedure may involve the use of simple random sampling (after stratification, where appropriate) at each of the two phases but it might often be more realistic to think of the first phase as being a simple random sample and the second phase coming from a Bernoulli process. In a survey of primary-care patients, for example, we might take a simple random sample of the patients registered in a given general practice, give them all a screening questionnaire and, finally, interview simple random samples from the screen-positives and the screen-negatives. In a study of people attending a primary-care clinic we might screen a series of consecutive attenders (loosely regarded as a simple random sample of all possible attenders), give them a screening questionnaire to complete on the spot, look at the results and then decide whether to interview immediately using a method equivalent to throwing a die.

We illustrate two-phase sampling by reference to two recent European surveys of psychiatric morbidity – one from Verona in northern Italy (Piccinelli *et al.*, 1995) and the other from Cantabria in northern Spain (Vázquez-Barquero *et al.*, 1997). The analysis of the former has been discussed in some detail by Dunn *et al.* (1999) and the latter by Pickles *et al.* (1995). In the first phase of the Verona survey 1558 subjects were asked to complete the GHQ-12 (Goldberg and Williams, 1988). These subjects were then stratified according to their GHQ score (low, medium or high) and sub-samples of these three strata then interviewed using the Composite International Diagnostic Interview – Primary-Care Version, the CIDI-PHC (see Von Korff and Üstün, 1995). Details of the second-phase data are given in Table 5.1. This survey has already been used as an illustration in Section 3.2 of the present book. In the first phase of the Cantabria survey the subjects were screened in two ways: the mental health status of the patients was determined through information provided by the general practitioner (GP) and the GHQ-28 (Goldberg and Williams, 1988). Patients were independently classified as being either GP+ (a case identified by the GP) or GP−, and as GHQ+ (a case identified by the GHQ using a score of 5 or over) or GHQ−. The screen-positives were defined by patients being GP+ or GHQ+, or both. Otherwise they were screen-negatives. Second-phase patients were then sub-sampled from these two strata and given a detailed psychiatric interview (see Vázquez-Barquero *et al.*, 1997, for full details). The results are shown in Table 5.2.

Table 5.1   Second-phase data from the Verona survey ($N = 250$)

Stratum 1 (GHQ 0–3): sampling weight $= 17.48$

	Sex		
	Male	Female	Total
Non-case	16	17	33
Case	8	19	27
			60

Stratum 2 (GHQ 4–5): sampling weight $= 4.94$

	Sex		
	Male	Female	Total
Non-case	9	5	14
Case	8	26	34
			48

Stratum 3 (GHQ >5): sampling weight $= 1.92$

	Sex		
	Male	Female	Total
Non-case	15	8	23
Case	28	91	119
			142

Estimate of overall prevalence: weighted number of cases/first-phase sample size

$$= [(27 \times 17.48) + (34 \times 4.94) + (119 \times 1.92)]/1558$$

$$= 0.56$$

Postscript In this section we have described the sampling procedures in terms of selection of the required samples from a known *finite* sampling frame. In practice this is often not available (consider the estimation of prevalence of depression in general practice attenders, for example), but even if it is we are not concerned with inferences about a particular finite population. We are more frequently interested in a potentially infinite *super-population* of potential attenders. For this reason the inferential procedures discussed below (standard error estimation, statistical modelling and construction of confidence intervals) do not refer to correction factors associated with sampling from finite populations. Readers who are unfamiliar with the literature on survey sampling statistics (see standard texts such as Cochran, 1977, or Lehtonen and Pahkinen, 1995) may not have noticed the apparent 'fudge' – but we mention it here, just in case!

Table 5.2   Second-phase data from the Cantabria survey ($N = 203$)

Stratum 1 (GHQ-negative and GP-negative): sampling weight = 12.24

	Sex		
	Male	Female	Total
Non-case	16	18	34
Case	2	6	8
			42

Stratum 2 (GHQ-positive or GP-positive, or both): sampling weight = 1.92

	Sex		
	Male	Female	Total
Non-case	19	58	77
Case	22	62	84
			161

Estimate of overall prevalence: weighted number of cases/first-phase sample size

$$= [(8 \times 12.24) + (84 \times 1.92)]/823$$
$$= 0.31$$

5.2   Estimation of prevalence

Suppose we have the results of a thorough diagnostic interview on 100 patients attending a general practice clinic (assume that these are, in fact, a simple random sample). We have found that 30 of them, say, were suffering from depression. The estimated prevalence of depression is 0.30. The standard error of this estimate is found by use of the formula in Table 5.3(a). The value is 0.046 and the corresponding 95% confidence interval for the prevalence of depression is approximately (0.21, 0.39). Now, suppose that this sample, instead of arising from simple random sampling, was actually a stratified sample: 70 women and 30 men (reflecting the proportions of women and men visiting the clinic). The stratum proportions are 70/100 (0.70) and 30/100 (0.30), respectively. Of the 70 women, 25 were depressed (prevalence estimate 0.36) and of the 30 men, five were depressed (prevalence estimate 0.17). The overall prevalence estimate is the weighted sum of the prevalences for women and men, using the stratum proportions as the weights. The prevalence estimate is 0.30, as before. But what is its standard error? This is found using the formula in Table 5.3(b). It is 0.045. The 95% confidence interval for the combined prevalence estimate is still (0.21, 0.39).

Finally, consider two-phase or double sampling. Suppose that the sample of 100 patients had initially been given a simple (and fallible) screening questionnaire to detect depression. Forty patients were classified as screen-positive and the other 60 screen-negative. The investigator now chose to interview all of

Table 5.3 Standard errors and 95% confidence intervals for estimated proportions

In all cases the 95% CI for a proportion, P, is approximated by

$$P - 1.96 \times \text{s.e.}(P) \quad \text{to} \quad P + 1.96 \times \text{s.e.}(P)$$

where the standard error, s.e.(P), depends on the sampling design as follows:

(a) Based on a simple random sample

Sample size:	N
Number with disease:	D
Estimated prevalence:	$P = D/N$
s.e.(P):	$\sqrt{\dfrac{P(1-P)}{N}}$

(b) Based on stratified sampling (with sample sizes proportional to strata sizes)

For Stratum i:

Stratum proportion (weight):	W_i
Sample size:	N_i
Number with disease:	D_i
Estimated prevalence:	$P_i = D_i/N_i$

Overall

Prevalence estimate, P:	$\Sigma_i W_i P_i$
s.e.(P):	$\sqrt{\Sigma\{W_i^2 P_i(1-P_i)/N_i\}}$

(c) Based on two-phase sampling (with two phase-one strata)

Total first-phase sample size:	N
Number screen-positive:	N_1
Proportion screen-positive:	W_1
Number screen-negative:	N_2
Proportion screen-negative:	W_2
Number of screen-positives in phase two:	M_1
Number diseased at phase two:	D_1
Proportion diseased:	$P_1 = D_1/M_1$
Number screen-negatives in phase two:	M_2
Number diseased at phase two:	D_2
Proportion diseased:	$P_2 = D_2/M_2$
Overall prevalence, P:	$W_1 P_1 + W_2 P_2$
s.e.(P):	$\sqrt{\begin{array}{l} W_1^2 P_1(1-P_1)/N_1 + W_2^2 P_2(1-P_2)/N_2 \\ \quad + (P_1 - P_2)^2 W_1 W_2/N \end{array}}$

the 40 screen-positives, but only 20 (33%) of the screen-negatives. Of the 40 screen-positives, 24 were found to be depressed on interview. Of the screen-negatives only two were found to be depressed on interview. Again, using the screen result as the stratification variable, the weighted sum of the two stratum prevalence estimates is 0.30, as before. The standard error (using the formula in Table 5.3(c) – allowing for the fact that the relative sizes of the two strata have been estimated rather than known *a priori*) is 0.056. The corresponding 95%

confidence interval is (0.19, 0.41). Note that the presumed gain in time and cost of not having to interview all of the screen-negative patients has only led to a marginal loss in the precision of the final prevalence estimate. Tables 5.1 and 5.2 illustrate the estimation of prevalence from the Verona and Cantabria studies, respectively, but estimation of standard errors from these data will be left for the time being.

Now let us approach the estimation problem from a slightly different perspective. In the new approach, which is mathematically equivalent to the one above and gives the same answers, we restrict the analysis to only those survey participants with complete data (that is, the second-phase subjects only). Information arising from the first-phase screen results and the second-phase sampling mechanism is provided by the assignment of a *sampling weight* to each individual subject, given by the inverse of the phase-two sampling fraction. For example, let us assume that we have a first-phase sample of 100 individuals who according to the screening questionnaire can be classified as likely cases (screen-positives) and likely non-cases (screen-negatives). Let us assume that we have found 60 of the latter. As above, in the second phase of the survey we interview 40 (i.e. 100%) of the likely cases and 20 (i.e. 33%) of the likely non-cases. The sampling weights corresponding to the phase-two subjects from the two strata are therefore 1 (i.e. 40/40) and 3 (i.e. 60/20), respectively. The sampling weight is an indicator of how many phase-one subjects are 'represented by' each of the phase-two records. Note that from here we work with data from the second-phase subjects only. There are data for 60 subjects $(40 + 20)$ and the sum of their sampling weights is 100 – that is, these 60 phase-two subjects represent the 100 $(40 \times 1 + 20 \times 3)$ phase-one subjects. Each phase-two subject is given an interview score of 1 if found to be a 'true' case; 0, otherwise. The sum of the products of this score and the sampling weights (i.e. $24 \times 1 + 2 \times 3$) gives the estimated number of first-phase 'true' cases represented by the 26 phase-two cases (i.e. 30). The obvious estimate of prevalence for the first-phase sample (and therefore the population from which it was drawn) is 30/100 or 30% (as before).

Now we will repeat the example of the use of sampling weights using algebraic notation. The symbol Σ will be used to denote summation across the second-phase data. Let $y_i = 1$ if the ith second-phase subject is a 'true' case, 0 otherwise. Let w_i be the ith subject's sampling weight. The estimate of the prevalence, π, is given by

$$\pi = \frac{\Sigma w_i y_i}{\Sigma w_i} \tag{5.1}$$

This is the well-known Horvitz–Thompson estimator from the sampling survey literature (see, for example, Lehtonen and Pahkinen, 1995), which has already been introduced in Chapter 3. The variance of π can be estimated through the use of the Taylor series expansion or through bootstrap sampling (see, for example, Pickles *et al.*, 1995; Clayton *et al.*, 1998). These methods can also provide large-sample confidence intervals for π. We will not discuss any technical details here but simply note that when using sampling weights great care should be used in the selection of appropriate statistical software (see Dunn *et al.*, 1999). Note, however, that the use of this method is quite straightforward even for quite complex stratification schemes for the second-phase sampling. In practice, it may be more convenient (and preferable from a theoretical point of view) to estimate prevalence via a weighted logistic regression model (by just fitting a constant term), produce a symmetrical confidence interval for the regression coefficient (i.e. the mean on the logistic scale), and then reverse the logistic transformation to produce the corresponding interval for the prevalence itself. The latter interval will not be symmetric about the point estimate but will always stay within the permitted range of a prevalence (0–100%) – see Section 3.2, where this approach has already been described. We discuss weighted logistic regression in more detail in the next section but here simply illustrate the method using the data from Verona and Cantabria (Tables 5.1 and 5.2, respectively).

Using the *Stata* logit command (see Appendix 5A) on the Verona results (together with sample or probability weights), we obtain an estimate of the logit of the prevalence of 0.230 (s.e. 0.187). The prevalence of psychiatric disorder is 56% (as in Table 5.1). The 95% confidence interval for the prevalence of disorder is (47%, 64%). Repeating the weighted logistic regression on the Cantabria data in *Stata* provides an estimate of the logit of the prevalence of −0.777 (prevalence = 31%, as in Table 5.2). The estimate of its standard error is 0.199. The 95% confidence interval for the prevalence of psychiatric disorder is (0.26, 0.40).

5.3 Weighted logistic regression models

The simplest modelling approach is an extension of the weighting estimation of prevalence, using sampling weights. The data are simply the second-phase interview results, relevant covariates and the appropriate sampling weights. The coefficients, β, of a logistic model are then estimated by maximising a modified form of the standard logistic log-likelihood that includes a sampling weight:

$$l(\beta) = \Sigma w_i \{ y_i x_i \beta + \log(1 - p_i) \} \qquad (5.2)$$

where y_i is the binary phase-two response, w_i is the corresponding sampling weight, p_i is the estimated response probability, and x_i is a vector of covariates.

The parameter covariance matrix (which is used to produce appropriate standard errors, confidence intervals and test statistics) is then obtained through the use of a robust information 'sandwich' or, alternatively, bootstrap sampling might be used to generate a robust parameter covariance matrix (see, for example, Binder, 1983, or Clayton *et al.*, 1998). The 'sandwich' estimator unrealistically treats the sampling weights as fixed. The bootstrap method, on the other hand, allows the weights to be a random variable. This is done by taking the bootstrap samples from the phase-one subjects, observing which of the subjects in the bootstrap sample have phase-two data and then recalculating the sampling weights. In practice the differences between the 'sandwich' and bootstrapped estimates of the standard error appears, in general, to be fairly trivial.

The above weighted logistic models when applied to those subjects with complete data only (i.e. the second-phase sample) may not be optimally efficient. If there have been covariates measured on subjects at phase one there are alternative, but technically more demanding, ways of modelling these data. Further details of alternative strategies for modelling two-phase data can be found in Pickles *et al.* (1995), Carroll *et al.* (1995) and Clayton *et al.* (1998). One way of getting extra efficiency from the straightforward weighted logistic models is through the careful choice of sampling weights. One preference is to use the *observed* sampling fraction to calculate the sampling weight, rather than that written into the design. If, for example, a Bernoulli sampling procedure was used in drawing the second-phase sample (planning to interview 50% of the screen-positive sub-sample from phase one) but, in fact, by chance we only obtained data from 30%, then it can be shown that it would be better to use the weight 100/30 in the analysis rather than 100/50 (Särndal *et al.*, 1992; Pepe *et al.*, 1994). Another improvement can be obtained (in the case of categorical predictors or covariates, at least) by calculating a separate sampling weight for each cell in the phase-two data. Subjects might be cross-classified by sex and age group, for instance, and in this case it might be advantageous to calculate sampling weights for each sex–age group combination (Pepe *et al.*, 1994). When we have a mix of categorical and quantitative covariates it might be useful to model sampling fractions using an (unweighted) logistic regression on the phase-one sample and then to use as the appropriate sampling weight for each phase-two subject the reciprocal of the response probability predicted by the model.

Returning to the Verona survey, the weighted prevalence estimates for men and women are 39.8% and 65.3%, respectively. We can use weighted logistic regression to compare the two sexes (by estimation of an odds-ratio or its natural logarithm). A direct estimate of the odds-ratio produced using the logistic command of *Stata* (using appropriate sampling weights) is 2.852 (s.e. 1.128). The 95% confidence interval for this odds-ratio is (1.314, 6.191). A similar analysis of the Spanish two-phase survey using *Stata* provides a 95% confidence interval for the above odds-ratio of (0.862, 4.738), the point estimate being 2.021 (s.e. 0.879). Appendix 5A provides the relevant *Stata* code.

5.4   Logistic models for multiple indicators of morbidity

In Chapter 4 we argued in favour of the use of multiple indicators. In fact, in a table such as Tables 5.1 and 5.2 we do have multiple indicators of psychiatric distress (two in the case of the Verona data, three in those from Cantabria). Our analysis so far, however, has not made use of this property. We have directed our attention to the interview results, treating the screening data as merely a way of making the design more efficient. But we could regard the screen and the diagnostic interview as a bivariate (or trivariate in the case of the Spanish data) response and model the data accordingly. Here the two types of response are treated symmetrically. We ask questions such as: what is the prevalence of illness according to the two indicators separately and what are the effects of social and demographic factors on prevalence according to the separate indicators? If there is an effect of sex, for example, it is then natural to ask if the effect of sex is the same for both of them or is there evidence of an indicator by sex interaction? If there is no statistically significant interaction then we might wish to constrain it to be zero and proceed to estimate the sex effect that is common to both indicators (this would be a more precise estimate than using either alone). The way to tackle these problems is through the use of multi-variate logistic regression – an approach that has been suggested by Fitzmaurice *et al.* (1995) and independently by Pickles *et al.* (1995). Fitzmaurice *et al.* were concerned with two indicators of childhood psychopathology (parental report and teacher's assessment) and made use of a full likelihood approach involving modelling the associations between the multiple indicators. We (Pickles *et al.*) were concerned with the use of screening questionnaires in multiphase sampling (the data in Table 5.2, in fact) and approached the problem as an extension of complex survey modelling. Here we explain the latter methods and leave the reader to consult Fitzmaurice *et al.* (1995) for the alternative.

From a survey sampling point of view, a multivariate analysis of both screen(s) and diagnostic interview implies a design in which these two (or more) responses (indicators) are nested by subject. Lavange *et al.* (1994) illustrate the application of survey logistic regression methods to repeated measurements on each subject. Software for the analysis of complex survey data (such as *SUDAAN* – Shah *et al.*, 1993 – or the survey and robust logistic regression procedures within *Stata*) allows one to accommodate clustering in the design of the survey (see cluster sampling in Section 5.1). Lavange *et al.* apply the same method to their repeated measures analyses by assuming that each subject corresponds to a cluster (using the terminology of the survey statistician, the *primary sampling unit* (PSU) is the subject, not the individual screen or interview result). In the case of data arising from two-phase samples we also, of course, have to make allowance for the observations that are missing within each cluster (subject) by design. Since screen responses are available for all subjects these receive expansion weights of 1, but responses on the diagnostic interview are weighted exactly as before (see Section 5.3). Although the responses will be correlated, ignoring this correlation will still yield consistent estimates of intercepts and slopes. Moreover, the parameter covariance matrix estimated using the Taylor series expansion method is robust to forms of model misspecification in the correlation among responses from within the same primary sampling unit (PSU). Thus this *independence working model* allows multivariate tests of effects. If we wish to use bootstrapping on data of this type we, again, have to remember to sample from phase one (not phase two) and also to sample the clusters or PSUs (subjects), not the individual within-subject records.

We illustrate this approach by examining the relative performance of the two screens (GHQ and GP) and diagnostic interview (SCAN) for the Cantabrian data in Table 5.2. Data on subjects from the second-phase sample comprise three records (corresponding to GHQ, GP and SCAN results) per subject (cluster or PSU). Data on subjects for which there is only first-phase information will comprise only two records (GHQ and GP results) per subject. Table 5.4

Table 5.4   Cantabrian data: percentage prevalence estimates (with their standard errors) for caseness determined by GHQ, GP and SCAN (weighted)

	GHQ	GP	SCAN
Men	24.69 (2.40)	11.42 (1.77)	22.31 (6.28)
Women	38.68 (2.18)	15.83 (1.63)	36.72 (5.55)
Odds-ratio	1.92 (0.30)	1.46 (0.31)	2.02 (0.88)
P-value	< 0.001	0.077	0.106
Both sexes combined	33.17 (1.64)	14.09 (1.21)	31.49 (4.28)

provides the required summary data. Clearly, the prevalence as determined from the view of the GP is much lower than that determined through the use of either the GHQ or the SCAN. The similarity of prevalence estimates obtained from the use of the GHQ and the SCAN should come as no surprise – the GHQ cut-off has been chosen so that it performs in the same way as the diagnostic interview. Irrespective of the choice of indicator, however, the prevalence is higher in men than in women (all three odds-ratios are greater than 1, but two of them do not reach statistical significance). Before we move on to fitting various models, note also that, as expected from the design, the standard errors of both the prevalence estimates and the odds-ratios are considerably higher for the interview data than that obtained using either screen.

If we were now to incorporate sex into a robust weighted logistic regression analysis we could explore the ways in which this characteristic differentially affects prevalence as identified by the three methods. If the three methods were distinguished by a within-subject factor called 'type' then this would involve the estimation and testing of the type by sex interaction. Here we use *Stata* to fit simple weighted logistic regression models for caseness as a function of type, sex and the type by sex interaction. For a similar analysis using *SUDAAN*, see Pickles *et al.* (1995) and Vázquez-Barquero *et al.* (1997). Appendix 5B gives the relevant *Stata* code. The *Stata* results are given in Table 5.5. We do not bother to present parameter estimates for the model including interaction terms as the latter did not differ significantly from zero. There is no convincing evidence that the sex effect is dependent on the method used as an indicator of psychiatric illness.

The effective use of weighted logistic regression is dependent on the assumption that the missing SCAN data are *ignorable* or, more specifically, *missing at random* (MAR) using the terminology of Little and Rubin (1987) – see Chapter 7 for

Table 5.5 Use of weighted logistic regression to compare multiple indicators of prevalence (using data from Table 5.2)

Model	Log-likelihood
(a) Type + Sex + Type × Sex	−1011.286
(b) Type + Sex	−1011.868
(c) Type	−1026.209
(d) Sex	−1050.065

Parameter estimates for model (b)

Effect*	Coefficient	Robust s.e.	P-value	Odds-ratio	95% C.I.
Sex (2)	0.613	0.198	0.002	1.846	1.251, 2.722
Type (2)	−1.123	0.106	<0.001	0.325	0.264, 0.401
Type (3)	−0.097	0.203	0.635	0.908	0.609, 1.352
Const.	−1.052	0.119			

* Interpretation of parameters: Sex (2) – women (Sex = 2) contrasted with men (Sex = 1); Type (2) – GP (Type = 2) contrasted with GHQ (Type = 1); Type(3) – SCAN (Type = 3) contrasted with GHQ (Type = 1)

further discussion of missing data problems. Here, we assume that there are no missing phase-one observations and that the only missing phase-two data arise from the use of the two-phase survey design. That is, we can assume that the probability of being part of the second-phase sample is dependent on the outcome of the first phase (the screening information provided by the GHQ and GP), but conditional on the screen response it is independent of the true state of the subject (that is the SCAN). Provided that the missing data mechanism is ignorable then there are a variety of estimation methods, including weighted logistic modelling, the use of GEE or full *maximum likelihood,* that yield consistent estimates. Further details can be found in Pickles *et al.* (1995) and in Pickles and Dunn (1998).

5.5   Appendix 5: *Stata* commands for two-phase survey data

A   Using only second-phase data

Using the Cantabrian phase-two data as an example, let us assume that we have data on the SCAN results (scan = 0 if −ve, 1 if +ve), screen status (screen = 0 if negative, 1 if positive), sex (1 = male; 2 = female) and corresponding sampling weights (w), as follows:

subject	scan	screen	sex	w
1	1	1	1	1.92
2	1	0	2	12.24
5	0	1	2	1.92
6	1	0	1	12.24
9	0	0	1	12.24
.	.	.		
.	.	.		
.	.	.		

(Note: subjects 3, 4, 7 and 8 did not receive a phase-two interview)

We can get an estimate of prevalence using

$$\text{svyprop scan [pweight} = \text{w]}$$

A corresponding logistic regression has the following form:

$$\text{logit scan [pweight} = \text{w]}$$

For separate estimates for each sex we can use:

$$\text{svyprop scan [pweight} = \text{w], by(sex)}$$

Logistic modelling can be carried out as follows:

$$\text{xi: logit scan i.sex [pweight} = \text{w]}$$

or

$$\text{xi: logistic scan i.sex [pweight} = \text{w]}$$

B   Using data from both phases in a repeated measures format

Suppose that we now have records corresponding to each of the three types of indicator:

subject	type	case	sex	w
1	1	1	1	1
1	2	1	1	1
1	3	1	1	1.92
2	1	0	2	1
2	2	0	2	1
2	3	0	2	12.24
3	1	0	2	1
3	2	0	2	1
4	1	1	1	1
4	2	1	1	1
5	1	1	2	1
5	2	1	2	1
5	3	1	2	1.92
.	.	.	.	.
.	.	.	.	.
.	.	.	.	.

Here, type (1 = GP, 2 = GHQ and 3 = SCAN) is a categorical variable to indicate which assessment method is being used. Case (0 = negative and 1 = positive) indicates whether the subject was given a positive diagnosis using the indicated method. As before, w is the sampling weight which is fixed at 1 for both the GP and the GHQ assessments, but is variable for the SCAN (= 1.92 for screen-positives and 12.24 for the negatives). Some subjects have three records (those who have both phase-one and phase-two data); others only have two (those with only phase-one data – i.e. they were not interviewed).

The appropriate logistic regression command is:

xi: logit case i.sex i.type [pweight = w], cluster(subject)

This fits the two main effects (sex being a between-subjects effect and type a within-subjects factor). To fit both main effects and an interaction use:

xi: logit case i.sex*i.type [pweight = w], cluster(subject)

6

Patterns of continuity and change

6.1 Introduction: a simple structural equation model

In this chapter we return to quantitative variables with measurement error and look at patterns of change in two illustrative areas: longitudinal panel studies and twin studies. Before proceeding, however, let us return to the GHQ data that was first presented in Table 2.1 and subsequently analysed using a confirmatory factor analysis model in Section 4.5. We use these data to illustrate a few basic ideas. We have data on the sum of the odd items and the even items of the GHQ-12 at two time points. Odd1 and Even1 are considered to be indicators of distress at time 1 and, similarly, Odd2 and Even2 are indicators of distress at time 2. In our factor analysis model we postulated two correlated latent variables, F_1 and F_2, corresponding to these two measures of distress, respectively. We now postulate a simple regression model to predict F_2 from F_1:

$$F_2 = \beta_f F_1 + D_2 \tag{6.1}$$

where β_f is the regression coefficient and D_2 the residual variation in F_2 that is not predicted by the linear relationship with F_1. Note that we are here only interested in analysing patterns of covariance and are therefore not concerned with the intercept term that is frequently found in a linear regression model. Equation (6.1) is an example of a simple *structural model*. Models such as these are often referred to as *causal models* but we avoid this terminology here because there is not necessarily any implication of causality and the issue of causality needs to treated with great care. An alternative term is *construct equation*. In addition to the construct equation described by (6.1) we have the four measurement equations as before:

$$
\begin{aligned}
\text{Odd1} &= \beta_e F_1 + E_1 \\
\text{Even1} &= \beta_e F_2 + E_2 \\
\text{Odd2} &= \beta_e F_1 + E_3 \\
\text{Even2} &= \beta_e F_2 + E_4
\end{aligned}
\tag{6.2}
$$

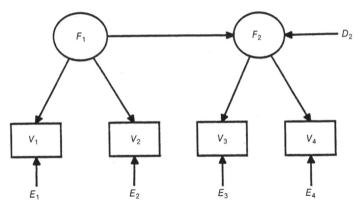

Figure 6.1 Path diagram for a structural equations model for GHQ scores.
Key:
F_1 – psychological distress at time 1
F_2 – psychological distress at time 2
V_1 – Odd1 (sum of odd items at time 1)
V_2 – Even1 (sum of even items at time 1)
V_3 – Odd2 (sum of odd items at time 2)
V_4 – Even2 (sum of even items at time 2)
E_1 to E_4 – disturbance terms associated with V_1 to V_4, respectively
D_2 – random disturbance term associated with F_2
Note: the single-headed arrow linking F_1 and F_2 indicates an implied direction of influence or causality.

with $\mathrm{Var}(E_1) = \mathrm{Var}(E_3) = \mathrm{Var}(E_2) = \mathrm{Var}(E_4) = \sigma_e^2$. The complete model is illustrated diagrammatically in Figure 6.1. As before, we specify that the variance of F_1 is 1. We do not, however, fix the variance of F_2 as this factor is now being predicted by F_1 and its variance is therefore given by

$$\mathrm{Var}(F_2) = \beta_f^2 \mathrm{Var}(F_1) + \mathrm{Var}(D_2)$$
$$= \beta_f^2 + \sigma_d^2 \qquad (6.3)$$

The expected covariance matrix is shown in Table 6.1(a). We fit the whole model to the covariance matrix using maximum likelihood. Appendix 6A illustrates the use of EQS for this. The resulting chi-square goodness-of-fit statistic is 10.789 with six degrees of freedom ($P = 0.095$). The estimates of β_e and σ_e^2 are 3.085 (s.e. 0.702) and 1.265 (s.e. 0.381), respectively. The corresponding estimates for the parameters of the construct equation, β_f and σ_d^2, are 0.917 (s.e. 0.138) and 0.067 (s.e. 0.093), respectively. Note that by constraining the variances or the errors (the Es) to be equal at the two times, but allowing the variance of F_2 to be estimated, we obtain differing estimates of reliability of the observed sub-scales at the two time points. These are obtained using the standardised estimates from the EQS output. At time 1 the reliability is $0.940^2 = 0.884$. At time 2 it is very slightly lower ($0.934^2 = 0.872$). β_f (i.e. 0.962) is an estimate of the *stability* of the latent psychological distress from one assessment to the next (note that it is time-dependent – if the intervals between assessments were to change so would the value of β_f). The proportion of the variation in F_2 that is 'explained' by F_1 is the square of the standardised estimate for β_f ($0.962^2 = 0.925$).

Table 6.1 Examples of expected covariance matrices

(a) Simple structural equations model for GHQ scores

	Odd1	Even1	Odd2	Even2
Odd1	$\beta_e^2 + \sigma_e^2$			
Even1	β_e^2	$\beta_e^2 + \sigma_e^2$		
Odd2	$\beta_e^2 \beta_f$	$\beta_e^2 \beta_f$	$(\beta_e \beta_f)^2 + \sigma_d^2 + \sigma_e^2$	
Even2	$\beta_e^2 \beta_f$	$\beta_e^2 \beta_f$	$(\beta_e \beta_f)^2 + \sigma_d^2$	$(\beta_e \beta_f)^2 + \sigma_d^2 + \sigma_e^2$

(b) The Wiley model for single indicator panel models

	V_1	V_2	V_3
V_1	$\sigma_f^2 + \sigma_e^2$		
V_2	$\beta \sigma_f^2$	$\beta^2 \sigma_f^2 + \sigma_d^2 + \sigma_e^2$	
V_3	$\beta^2 \sigma_f^2$	$\beta^3 \sigma_f^2 + \beta \sigma_d^2$	$\beta^4 \sigma_f^2 + (\beta^2 + 1)\sigma_d^2 + \sigma_e^2$

6.2 Autoregressive models for single-indicator panel data

The GHQ data described in the above section can be thought of as arising from a two-indicator two-wave *panel study*. Basically, a panel is a particular type of *cohort* in which the subjects are assessed at two or more discrete times – the intervals between the repeated assessments usually being of equal size. The simplest panel study involves a single assessment on each of two occasions (a test–retest reliability study, for example). The above GHQ example illustrates a two-indicator two-wave panel study. In the present section we will introduce statistical models for single-indicator panel data. The aim of collecting this type of data is usually to enable us to separate out the effects of measurement imprecision (lack of reliability) and instability.

When we have a single fallible indicator at each of two time points (a test–retest reliability study) then it is impossible to distinguish measurement error from lack of stability of the underlying latent variable that we wish to measure – the two are completely confounded. If we have measurements available at three or more occasions, however, we can make progress. An early attempt at separating reliability and stability was made by Heise (1969). A more realistic solution was provided by Wiley and Wiley (1970), and it is this that will form the basis of the present discussion. The Wiley model is essentially a first-order *autoregressive* (or *simplex*) *model* for the latent variable under consideration. Consider a panel study in which every subject provides three repeated measurements V_1, V_2 and V_3. The time interval between V_1 and V_2 may or may not be equal to that between V_2 and V_3. We postulate the three following measurement equations:

$$V_1 = F_1 + E_1$$
$$V_2 = F_2 + E_2 \qquad (6.4)$$
$$V_3 = F_3 + E_3$$

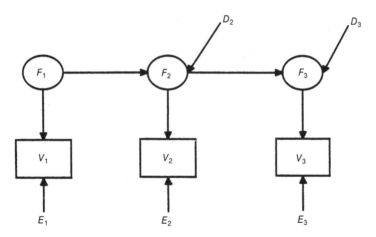

Figure 6.2   Path diagram for the Wiley model for children's depression scores.
Key:
F_1 – depression at time 1
F_2 – depression at time 2
F_3 – depression at time 3
V_1 – CDI score at time 1
V_2 – CDI score at time 2
V_3 – CDI score at time 3
E_1 to E_3 – disturbance terms associated with V_1 to V_3, respectively
D_2 and D_3 – random disturbance terms associated with F_2 and F_3, respectively.

F_1, F_2 and F_3 are the values of the latent variable at each of the three time points and E_1, E_2 and E_3 are the corresponding measurement errors. We assume that the errors are uncorrelated with both the latent variables and with each other. We now assume that F_2 is linearly related to, but not necessarily the same as, F_1. Similarly, F_3 is linearly related to F_2. The *partial correlation* between F_3 and F_1, given F_2, is however assumed to be zero. These assumptions are expressed in the following two construct equations:

$$F_2 = \beta_2 F_1 + D_2$$
$$F_3 = \beta_3 F_2 + D_3 \tag{6.5}$$

The combination of the measurement equations (6.3) and construct equations (6.4) is illustrated graphically in Figure 6.2.

We can again use software such as EQS to fit the expected covariance matrix to appropriate data and estimate the various parameters (see Appendix 6B). Before doing this, however, we have to introduce some constraints to make the model identified. Wiley and Wiley assumed that the variance of the measurement errors (the Es) was constant over time – let this common variance be σ_e^2. The variance of F_1 is free to be estimated (σ_f^2), but those of F_2 and F_3 are determined by the construct equations. Note, again, that constant measurement error variance does not imply constant reliability. In the example that we are about to use the time intervals between the repeated assessments are equal and we will therefore assume that both $\beta_2 = \beta_3 (= \beta$, say) and $Var(D_2) = Var(D_3) = \sigma_d^2$. The variance

Table 6.2 Covariance and correlation matrices for three successive assessments of depression in 330 children (covariances calculated using data on correlations from Cole *et al.*, 1998)

(a) Covariance matrix

	CDI1	CDI2	CDI3
CDI1	60.840		
CDI2	46.164	67.568	
CDI3	43.110	50.040	64.160

(b) Correlations

	CDI1	CDI2	CDI3
CDI1	1.00		
CDI2	0.72	1.00	
CDI3	0.69	0.76	1.00

σ_e^2 is a measure of lack of precision whereas σ_d^2 reflects lack of stability. To summarise, the model defines the expected covariance which has the form shown in Table 6.1(b).

Wiley and Wiley (1970) defined stability coefficients, γ_{jk}, as the correlation between latent factors at times j and k. Direct estimates can be obtained using the standardised β values (β^*, say) as available from EQS output, for example. From our simplifying constraints, it follows that both γ_{12} and γ_{13} are equal to β_2^* and β_3^*, respectively (remembering that equality constraints on unstandardised β coefficients do not imply the equivalent constraints after they have been standardised. γ_{13} is equal to the product $\beta_2^* \beta_3^*$.

Table 6.2 provides an observed correlation matrix and corresponding covariance matrix for three successive, equally spaced (the interval between waves being six months), self-reported measures of depression in children and adolescents (extracted from a much larger table in Cole *et al.*, 1998). The depression scores were obtained using the Children's Depression Inventory (CDI; Kovacs, 1981). Fitting the above model to these data provides a chi-square of 3.088 with two degrees of freedom ($P = 0.214$). The estimated value of β is 0.961 (s.e. 0.040) and that for σ_d^2 is 6.178 (s.e. 3.111). The estimates of σ_f^2 and σ_e^2 are 47.96 (s.e. 5.032) and 13.678 (s.e. 2.107), respectively, implying a reliability for V_1 of 0.778. Inspection of the standardised solution (see Table 6.3(a)) reveals reliabilities for V_1, V_2 and V_3 of 0.778 (0.882^2), 0.787 (0.887^2) and 0.794 (0.891^2), respectively. Standardised estimates of the coefficient β provide indicators of stability between times 1 and 2 (0.937) and between times 2 and 3 (0.940). That for times 1 and 3 is the product of these two estimates.

Table 6.4 gives the correlation and covariance matrices for assessments of depression and anxiety for the above three assessments (again, this has been extracted from a much larger table from Cole *et al.*, 1998). The covariance of depression and anxiety scores will be discussed in the next section. Here we have a look at a simple autoregressive model for the anxiety measures. These have been obtained using the Revised Children's Manifest Anxiety Scale (RCMAS; Reynolds and Richmond, 1978). Fitting the above model to the

Table 6.3 Standardised solution for the Wiley model (using data from Cole et al., 1998)

(a) For depression scores*

$$CDI1 = V_1 = 0.882F_1 + 0.471E_1$$
$$CDI2 = V_2 = 0.887F_2 + 0.462E_2$$
$$CDI3 = V_3 = 0.891F_3 + 0.454E_3$$

$$DEP2 = F_2 = 0.937F_1 + 0.350D_2$$
$$DEP3 = F_3 = 0.940F_2 + 0.342D_3$$

(b) For anxiety scores*

$$RCMAS1 = V_1 = 0.904F_1 + 0.427E_1$$
$$RCMAS2 = V_2 = 0.907F_2 + 0.422E_2$$
$$RCMAS3 = V_3 = 0.908F_3 + 0.418E_3$$

$$ANX2 = F_2 = 0.923F_1 + 0.386D_2$$
$$ANX3 = F_3 = 0.925F_2 + 0.381D_3$$

* DEP2 and DEP3 are the latent variables for depression at time 2 and time 3, respectively; ANX2 and ANX3 are the corresponding latent variables for anxiety.

anxiety data yields a chi-square of 6.176 with two degrees of freedom ($P = 0.046$). The model does not fit quite so well but we will assume that it provides an adequate description of the data. The standardised solution for the parameter estimates is provided in Table 6.3(b). The anxiety measures appear to be slightly more reliable than those for depression, but marginally less stable.

Table 6.4 Covariance and correlation matrices for three successive assessments of both depression and anxiety in 330 children (covariances calculated using data on correlations from Cole et al., 1998)

(a) Covariance matrix

	CDI1	RCMAS1	CDI2	RCMAS2	CDI3	RCMAS3
CDI1	60.840					
RCMAS1	64.701	140.422				
CDI2	46.164	56.496	67.568			
RCMAS2	55.638	104.585	70.560	146.168		
CDI3	43.110	54.104	50.040	63.915	64.160	
RCMAS3	56.620	98.710	64.560	113.658	74.349	141.610

(b) Correlations

	CDI1	RCMAS1	CDI2	RCMAS2	CDI3	RCMAS3
CDI1	1.00					
RCMAS1	0.70	1.00				
CDI2	0.72	0.58	1.00			
RCMAS2	0.59	0.73	0.71	1.00		
CDI3	0.69	0.57	0.76	0.66	1.00	
RCMAS3	0.61	0.70	0.66	0.79	0.78	1.00

6.3 Models for multiple-indicator multiwave panel data

Now consider panel data in which several indicators are utilised for each wave. They might all be measures of the same concept, or they might measure different things (or both). We will illustrate some of the approaches to the analysis of this type of data by reference to the relatively simple covariance matrix in Table 6.4. Here each child has a single measure of depression and a single measure of anxiety, both available at each of the three waves of the study. We have already looked at simple autoregressive models for depression and anxiety separately; we now consider models for both together.

We start by assuming that the separate autoregressive models for depression and anxiety also hold when we study both simultaneously. Our main concern here is to describe the relationships between the changing measurement of depression and anxiety. Does anxiety influence depression, for example, or the other way round? Does anxiety at time 2 directly influence depression at time 2, or is the second depression factor more influenced by anxiety at the previous time point? Because of identifiability problems, we are limited in the number of options that we can pursue. First, we assume that there are two independent (in the sense used in a regression model) latent variables (apart from residuals or error terms) in the model: a depression factor at time 1 and a corresponding factor for anxiety. The two factors are correlated. We then model the factors for depression and anxiety at the following times (i.e. waves two and three) as variables that are in some way dependent on the initial

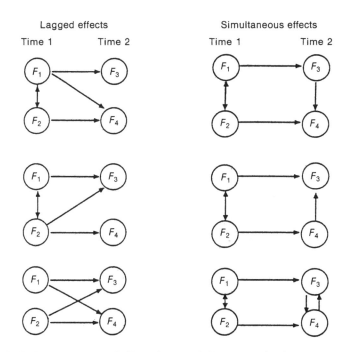

Figure 6.3   Different patterns of effect of two variables on each other.

values (as in the case of the earlier autoregressive models, in fact). We assume that there are no direct links between measures at time 1 and those at time 2 (i.e. we keep our assumption that the partial correlation between any time 1 measure and any time 3 measure is zero, conditional on measurements at time 2. The effects that we can now test and estimate are either between variables measured at the same time (e.g. is DEP2 predicted from ANX2?) or between variables measured at adjacent time points (is DEP2 predicted directly by ANX1, for example?). Note that it does not make sense in this context to ask whether variables measured early in the data set might be influenced by those measured at the next wave. The possible patterns of the effects of the two time 1 factors on each of the time 2 factors are illustrated by the path diagrams in Figure 6.3. Basically the effects can be assumed to be either *lagged* (the left-hand diagrams) or *simultaneous* (the right-hand ones). In their analyses, Cole *et al.* (1998) appeared to be primarily concerned with cross-lagged effects. We start by fitting the equivalent of the model in the bottom left-hand corner of Figure 6.3. It is presented in Table 6.5 and illustrated graphically in Figure 6.4. The main points to note are that (a) the measurement models are constrained to

Table 6.5 Cross-lagged panel model for depression and anxiety

(a) Measurement equations

$$
\begin{aligned}
V_1 &= \quad \text{CDI1} = F_1 (= \text{DEP1}) + E_1 \\
V_2 &= \text{RCMAS1} = F_2 (= \text{ANX1}) + E_2 \\
V_3 &= \quad \text{CDI2} = F_3 (= \text{DEP2}) + E_3 \\
V_4 &= \text{RCMAS2} = F_4 (= \text{ANX2}) + E_4 \\
V_5 &= \quad \text{CDI3} = F_5 (= \text{DEP3}) + E_5 \\
V_6 &= \text{RCMAS3} = F_6 (= \text{ANX3}) + E_6
\end{aligned}
$$

(b) Construct equations

$$
\begin{aligned}
\text{DEP2} &= F_3 = \beta_1 F_1 + \beta_2 F_2 + D_3 \\
\text{ANX2} &= F_4 = \beta_3 F_1 + \beta_4 F_2 + D_4 \\
\text{DEP3} &= F_5 = \beta_1 F_1 + \beta_2 F_2 + D_5 \\
\text{ANX3} &= F_6 = \beta_3 F_1 + \beta_4 F_2 + D_6
\end{aligned}
$$

(c) Estimated variances

$$\text{Var}(F_1), \text{Var}(F_2), \text{Var}(E_1) \text{ to } \text{Var}(E_6), \text{Var}(D_3) \text{ to } \text{Var}(D_6)$$

(d) Estimated covariances

$$\text{Cov}(F_1, F_2), \text{Cov}(E_1, E_2), \text{Cov}(E_3, E_4), \text{Cov}(E_5, E_6)$$

(e) Constraints (other than those implied by the numbering of the βs)

$$
\begin{aligned}
\text{Var}(E_1) &= \text{Var}(E_3) = \text{Var}(E_5) \\
\text{Var}(E_2) &= \text{Var}(E_4) = \text{Var}(E_6) \\
\text{Cov}(E_1, E_2) &= \text{Cov}(E_3, E_4) = \text{Cov}(E_5, E_6) \\
\text{Var}(D_3) &= \text{Var}(D_5) \\
\text{Var}(D_4) &= \text{Var}(D_6)
\end{aligned}
$$

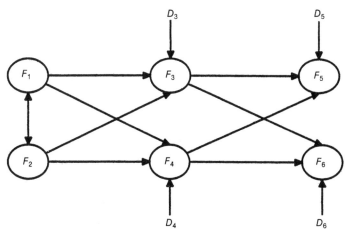

Figure 6.4   Path diagram for model with lagged effects for children's depression and anxiety scores (excluding observed variables for simplicity).
Key:
F_1 – depression at time 1
F_2 – anxiety at time 1
F_3 – depression at time 2
F_4 – anxiety at time 2
F_5 – depression at time 3
F_6 – anxiety at time 3
D_3 to D_6 – random disturbance terms associated with F_3 to F_6, respectively.

have the same parameter values at each of the three time points (we have allowed measurement errors for depression and anxiety to be correlated), and (b) the construct equations describing the changes from time 2 to time 3 are the same as those for time 1 to time 2 and the corresponding regression coefficients and variances of the residuals (the Ds) have accordingly been constrained to be equal for the two time intervals. Fitting this model using maximum likelihood (see Appendix 6C) gives a chi-square of 20.595 based on nine degrees of freedom ($P = 0.015$). The fit is not particularly good (although other goodness-of-fit indices such as the Bentler–Bonett indices (0.99) – see Bentler, 1995; Dunn, Everitt and Pickles, 1993 – suggest that it might be good enough). The standardised estimates are given in Table 6.6. The unstandardised estimate of β_2 (the effect of anxiety at time i on depression at time $i + 1$) is 0.045 (s.e. 0.047). The estimate of β_4 (the effect of depression at time i on anxiety at time $i + 1$) is 0.270 (s.e. 0.097).

If, instead of fitting the cross-lagged effects as estimated by β_2 and β_4 in the above model, we now fit simultaneous effects (as illustrated by Figure 6.5) then we get a model that fits just as well (or, in fact, slightly better). The resulting chi-square is 18.487 with nine degrees of freedom ($P = 0.030$). The Bentler–Bonett fit indices are unchanged (0.99). If β_2 now reflects the simultaneous effect of anxiety on depression then its unstandardised estimate is 0.082 (s.e. 0.045). The simultaneous effect of depression on anxiety (β_4) is 0.291 (s.e. 0.090). The full standardised solution is given in Table 6.7. Which of the two

Table 6.6   Standardised solution for the cross-lagged model for anxiety and depression (using data from Cole *et al.*, 1998)

(a) The measurement equations

$$CDI1 = V_1 = 0.854F_1 + 0.521E_1$$
$$RCMAS1 = V_2 = 0.882F_2 + 0.471E_2$$
$$CDI2 = V_3 = 0.859F_3 + 0.511E_3$$
$$RCMAS2 = V_4 = 0.884F_4 + 0.467E_4$$
$$CDI3 = V_5 = 0.865F_5 + 0.501E_5$$
$$RCMAS3 = V_6 = 0.888F_6 + 0.460E_6$$

(b) The construct equations

$$DEP2 = F_3 = 0.933F_1 + 0.068F_2 + 0.350D_2$$
$$ANX2 = F_4 = 0.829F_2 + 0.172F_1 + 0.262D_4$$
$$DEP3 = F_5 = 0.932F_3 + 0.066F_4 + 0.165D_5$$
$$ANX3 = F_6 = 0.821F_4 + 0.173F_3 + 0.257D_6$$

models is the better? It is almost impossible to make a safe decision. The fit of the second one (simultaneous effects) is a marginal improvement on the first (cross-lagged effects) but, on the other hand, the simultaneous effects model appears to explain less of the variability of the latent dependent variables (as indicated by the size of the standardised effects associated with D_3 to D_6).

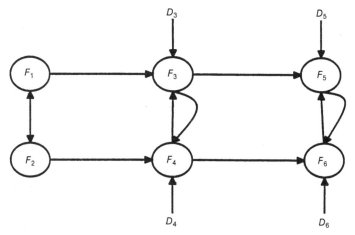

Figure 6.5   Path diagram for model with simultaneous effects for children's depression and anxiety scores (excluding observed variables for simplicity).
Key:
F_1 – depression at time 1
F_2 – anxiety at time 1
F_3 – depression at time 2
F_4 – anxiety at time 2
F_5 – depression at time 3
F_6 – anxiety at time 3
D_3 to D_6 – random disturbance terms associated with F_3 to F_6, respectively.

Table 6.7   Standardised solution for the model for anxiety and depression with simultaneous effects (using data from Cole *et al.*, 1998)

(a) The measurement equations

$$CDI1 = V_1 = 0.873F_1 + 0.488E_1$$
$$RCMAS1 = V_2 = 0.894F_2 + 0.448E_2$$
$$CDI2 = V_3 = 0.878F_3 + 0.479E_3$$
$$RCMAS2 = V_4 = 0.896F_4 + 0.444E_4$$
$$CDI3 = V_5 = 0.883F_5 + 0.469E_5$$
$$RCMAS3 = V_6 = 0.900F_6 + 0.437E_6$$

(b) The construct equations

$$DEP2 = F_3 = 0.855F_1 + 0.124F_4 + 0.291D_2$$
$$ANX2 = F_4 = 0.794F_2 + 0.191F_3 + 0.314D_4$$
$$DEP3 = F_5 = 0.854F_3 + 0.123F_6 + 0.283D_5$$
$$ANX3 = F_6 = 0.787F_4 + 0.193F_5 + 0.308D_6$$

The moral is that you should not simply rely on a single model that appears to fit the data. Try to think of all the other possibilities – there might be other models that fit just as well or even better than the one you thought of first.

6.4   A measurement model for twin data

We now move on from the investigation of patterns of stability over time to continuity within families and, in particular, the shared characteristics of twins. We start by considering a common measurement model for data collected on two groups of subjects: identical or *monozygotic* (*MZ*) *twins* and the corresponding non-identical or *dizygotic* (*DZ*) *twins*. The data we use to illustrate the method come from Hewitt *et al.* (1992). These authors were concerned with a genetic model for parental ratings of their own children's behaviour problems. To make life relatively simple we restrict our analysis of data to that from young boys (see Table 6.8). We also restrict our discussion to one of several different measurement models. Readers who wish to explore this area further are referred to Hewitt *et al.* (1992) or Simonoff *et al.* (1995) for further information. In this section we are essentially concerned with the estimation of the correlation between the *latent phenotypes* of both the MZ and the DZ twins. That is, we aim to look at the similarity of the twin pairs after allowing for attenuation due to measurement errors. We will, however, also have a look at the reliability of the parents' ratings and also see that they have a tendency to overestimate the resemblance between their offspring. We have used the word 'overestimate' in a slightly off-hand manner, however. In the modelling below we treat the raised estimation of twin resemblance as arising from a correlated measurement error. This is not necessarily the case, however, as the increased similarity observed by one parent might arise from the fact that they are observing behaviour not witnessed by the other parent or any of the other observers (including the twins themselves). After consideration of the measurement

Table 6.8   Observed covariance/correlation matrix for parental ratings of the behaviour of young male twins (from Hewitt *et al.*, 1992). Variances are on the diagonal, covariances are below it and the correlations are above

(a) Monozygotic (MZ) twins

| | Twin 1 | | Twin 2 | |
	Mother (MT1)	Father (FT1)	Mother (MT2)	Father (FT2)
MT1	0.694	0.47	0.84	0.46
FT1	0.312	0.638	0.37	0.72
MT2	0.569	0.238	0.666	0.45
FT2	0.308	0.461	0.293	0.647

(b) Dizygotic (DZ) twins

| | Twin 1 | | Twin 2 | |
	Mother (MT1)	Father (FT1)	Mother (MT2)	Father (FT2)
MT1	0.565	0.41	0.55	0.29
FT1	0.241	0.604	0.25	0.57
MT2	0.291	0.137	0.488	0.52
FT2	0.171	0.347	0.285	0.604

model generating the latent phenotypes we will then move on (in the following section) to think about further modelling to explain the resulting pattern of correlation between these latent phenotypes.

The labelling of the two twins as twin 1 and twin 2 is usually quite arbitrary and is frequently determined by the order in which they (or their parents) provide information. This ought to be decided in advance as a randomised part of the design of the data collection procedures. For each twin we have a mother's rating of behaviour and a corresponding rating from the father. We start by assuming that each parent is assessing a common latent phenotype (labelled as F_1 in twin 1 and F_2 in twin 2).

The by now familiar measurement equations are given in Table 6.9. F_1 and F_2 are both constrained to have a variance of unity. We assume that the same measurement model holds for each of the two twins and constrains all relevant parameter estimates to be the same for the two twins. Table 6.9 should clarify this. We now use EQS to simultaneously fit the measurement equations to both groups of twins, constraining all parameter estimates to be the same in the two groups except for the correlation between the latent phenotypes F_1 and F_2 (i.e. these are ρ_{mz} and ρ_{dz} for MZ twins and DZ twins, respectively). Appendix 6D illustrates the EQS program for doing this (but, to be precise, it is the program for fitting the modified model allowing for correlated errors – see below). If we assume that the four measurement errors are all mutually uncorrelated then we obtain a very poor fit (chi-square = 97.983 with 14 degrees of freedom; $P = 0.001$). We now modify the model to enable the mother's ratings for the twins to be correlated. We also allow a similar correlation for the two father ratings. These two modifications are allowing both the mothers

Table 6.9   Factor model for parental ratings of the behaviour of young male twins

(a)   Measurement equations

$$V_1 = \text{MT1} = \beta_1 F_1 (= \text{PHE1}) + E_1$$
$$V_2 = \text{FT1} = \beta_2 F_1 (= \text{PHE1}) + E_2$$
$$V_3 = \text{MT2} = \beta_1 F_2 (= \text{PHE2}) + E_3$$
$$V_4 = \text{FT22} = \beta_2 F_2 (= \text{PHE2}) + E_4$$

(b)   Estimated variances

$$\text{Var}(E_1) \text{ to } \text{Var}(E_4)$$

(c)   Estimated covariances

$$\text{Cov}(F_1, F_2) = \rho, \text{Cov}(E_1, E_3), \text{Cov}(E_2, E_4)$$

(d)   Within-group constraints (other than those implied by the numbering of the βs)

$$\text{Var}(E_1) = \text{Var}(E_3)$$
$$\text{Var}(E_2) = \text{Var}(E_4)$$

and the fathers to independently 'overestimate' the similarity between their twin children. The model is equivalent to the *Rater Bias Model* of Hewitt *et al.* (1992). The resulting chi-square is now 9.003 with 12 degrees of freedom ($P = 0.703$). The parameter estimates are given in Table 6.10. Note that the reliability

Table 6.10   Factor analysis model for parental ratings of the behaviour of young male twins (data from Hewitt *et al.*, 1992)

(a) Parameter estimates

Parameter	Estimate	Standard error
β_1	0.655	0.106
β_2	0.425	0.072
$\sigma_1^2 \ (= \sigma_3^2)$	0.164	0.133
$\sigma_2^2 \ (= \sigma_4^2)$	0.440	0.067
σ_{13}	0.096	0.110
σ_{24}	0.266	0.059
ρ_{mz}	0.902	0.053
ρ_{dz}	0.591	0.102

(b) Standardised solution

$$\text{MT1} = V_1 = 0.851 F_1 + 0.526 E_1$$
$$\text{FT1} = V_2 = 0.539 F_1 + 0.842 E_1$$
$$\text{MT2} = V_3 = 0.851 F_2 + 0.526 E_1$$
$$\text{FT2} = V_4 = 0.539 F_2 + 0.842 E_1$$

of the mothers' ratings ($= 0.851^2$) appears to be considerably higher than those of the fathers ($= 0.539^2$). Note that, although the covariance for the mothers' measurement errors for the two twins ($\sigma_{13} = 0.096$) is considerably less than the corresponding covariance for the fathers ($\sigma_{24} = 0.266$), the measurement error correlations for mothers and fathers are actually very similar (0.587 and 0.605, respectively). The covariances are different because of the relative lack of precision of the fathers' ratings.

Finally, let us have a look at the correlation between the latent phenotypes of the twins. For the MZ twins the estimate (ρ_{mz}) is 0.902. The corresponding figure for the DZs (ρ_{dz}) is 0.591. As expected, MZ twins reveal more similarity than their DZ counterparts. These estimates should be compared with the correlations that have not been corrected for attenuation due to measurement error. From Table 6.8 we can see that the correlations for the mothers' ratings are 0.84 and 0.55 for MZs and DZs, respectively. The corresponding correlations for the fathers' ratings are 0.72 and 0.57, respectively. There appears to be evidence that the propensity to display behaviour problems is inherited.

6.5   The ACE model with measurement error

It is beyond the scope of the present text to go into a detailed discussion of biometrical genetics. For that the reader is referred to the book by Sham (1998). We will simply assume (without justification) that the latent phenotype of an individual arises from three independent components. These are an *A*dditive genetic component, a *C*ommon environmental component and a specific *E*nvironmental component (hence the *ACE model*). The common environmental component comprises those non-genetic influences that have been shared by the two twins whereas the specific environmental component comprises those influences or experiences that are unique to each of the two twins. The ACE model can then be represented by the following construct equations:

$$F_1 = \beta_3 F_3 + \beta_4 F_4 + D_1$$
$$F_2 = \beta_3 F_5 + \beta_4 F_4 + D_2$$

(6.6)

where F_3 and F_5 are the additive genetic factors for twin 1 and twin 2, respectively. From genetic theory we would expect that the correlation between F_3 and F_5 should be 1.0 in MZ twins but 0.5 in DZs. F_4 is the environmental factor that is common to both twins. Finally, D_1 and D_2 are random disturbance terms representing their specific environment. They are uncorrelated with each other but are constrained to have a common variance. The full model (including the required measurement equations and constraints) is illustrated in Table 6.11. The program to fit this model in EQS is shown in Appendix 6E. The resulting chi-square is 9.003 with 12 degrees of freedom. This is exactly the same as the final model from Section 6.4. Why? Basically it is because it is an equivalent model (it has the same number of estimated parameters, for example) and we are simply partitioning the variance of the

Table 6.11   ACE model for parental ratings of the behaviour of young male twins

---

(a) Measurement equations

$$V_1 = \text{MT1} = \beta_1 F_1 (= \text{PHE1}) + E_1$$
$$V_2 = \text{FT1} = \beta_2 F_1 (= \text{PHE1}) + E_2$$
$$V_3 = \text{MT2} = \beta_1 F_2 (= \text{PHE2}) + E_3$$
$$V_4 = \text{FT2} = \beta_2 F_2 (= \text{PHE2}) + E_4$$

(b) Construct equations (the ACE model)

$$F_1 = \beta_3 F_3 (= \text{ADD}) + \beta_4 F_4 (= \text{CENV}) + D_1$$
$$F_2 = \beta_3 F_5 (= \text{ADD}) + \beta_4 F_4 (= \text{CENV}) + D_2$$

(c) Estimated variances

$$\text{Var}(E_1) \text{ to Var}(E_4), \text{Var}(D_1), \text{Var}(D_2)$$

(d) Estimated covariances

$$\text{Cov}(E_1, E_3), \text{Cov}(E_2, E_4)$$

(e) Within-group constraints (other than those implied by the numbering of the βs)

$$\text{Var}(E_1) = \text{Var}(E_3)$$
$$\text{Var}(E_2) = \text{Var}(E_4)$$
$$\text{Var}(D_1) = \text{Var}(D_2)$$
$$\text{Cov}(F_3, F_5) = 1.0 \text{ in MZ twins}$$
$$\text{Cov}(F_3, F_5) = 0.50 \text{ in DZ twins}$$

---

twins' phenotype into its three components. In our earlier model we have already constrained the total variation to be the same in both MZ and DZ twins. We are now introducing a particular pattern to explain the relative sizes of ρ_{mz} and ρ_{dz}. Although we are estimating three new parameters (β_3, β_4 and σ_D^2), these are replacing the separate estimates of ρ_{mz} and ρ_{dz}. We still appear to be estimating one more parameter, however, but if we look carefully at the contents of Appendix 6E we will see that we have fixed the value of β_1 to be 1.0. This restriction is a necessary introduction to retain model identifiability.

The required parameter estimates are given in Table 6.12. As would be expected from the above discussion there are no changes to the measurement equation parameters. The relative proportions of the variability in the latent phenotype that is explained by additive genetic variation, common environmental and specific environmental components are obtained from the standardised solution. They are 0.623 ($= 0.789^2$), 0.281 ($= 0.530^2$) and 0.097 ($= 0.312^2$), respectively.

Before we leave this section let us briefly revisit the finding that the ACE model for the latent phenotype (as fitted in this section) is exactly equivalent to the measurement model in Section 6.4. Our modelling cannot be used to

Table 6.12   ACE model for parental ratings of the behaviour of young male twins (data from Hewitt *et al.*, 1992)

(a) Parameter estimates

Parameter	Estimate	Standard error
β_2	0.649	0.192
β_3	0.517	0.072
β_4	0.347	0.168
σ_D^2	0.042	0.030
$\sigma_1^2\ (=\sigma_3^2)$	0.164	0.133
$\sigma_2^2\ (=\sigma_4^2)$	0.440	0.067
σ_{13}	0.096	0.110
σ_{24}	0.266	0.059

(b) Standardised solution

$$MT1 = V_1 = 0.850F_1 + 0.526E_1$$
$$FT1 = V_2 = 0.539F_1 + 0.842E_1$$
$$MT2 = V_3 = 0.850F_2 + 0.526E_1$$
$$FT2 = V_4 = 0.539F_2 + 0.842E_1$$

$$PHE1 = F_1 = 0.789F_3 + 0.530F_4 + 0.312D_1$$
$$PHE2 = F_2 = 0.789F_3 + 0.530F_4 + 0.312D_2$$

justify the ACE model for the latent phenotype but merely as a way of estimating the contributions of the three components.

6.6   General modelling strategies

In psychiatric epidemiology, as in any other area of epidemiology, we are often searching for apparent causes or explanations for variations in illness or distress. Following the influential work of Brown and Harris (1978) on depression, for example, we may be interested in risk factors such as stress and adverse life events and the protective or buffering effects of social support. Such *stress-buffering models* have an extensive literature and the reader is referred to Wheaton (1985) for a detailed discussion of many of the statistical issues. But life is a bit complicated: 'Although life events may previously have been considered as chance occurrences and unpleasant events to reflect bad luck, it has increasingly been recognised that the relationship between individuals and their environment is an interactive one' (Thapar and McGuffin, 1996). A simple causal link from environmental risk to illness is obviously unrealistic. People's personalities influence whether they might be at greater or lesser risk of illness, and their personalities also have an influence on their choice (or otherwise) of social and physical environment. Twin studies have shown that depression and many other psychiatric problems have a genetic component (see, for example Dunn, Everitt and Pickles, 1993) but so apparently have both reported stressful life events (Plomin *et al.*, 1990; Kendler *et al.*, 1993; Thapar and McGuffin, 1996) and social support (Plomin, 1994). Sorting out all the environmental and genetic risk factors and the potentially complex interactions between them is no simple task. We will make no attempt to do so here or even attempt to explain how it might be done. There are two things to reiterate at this point, however. The first is that all indicators of psychiatric or behavioural distress and most of the indicators of risk are subject to measurement error. This fact is ignored by the investigator at her peril. The second is that the investigator should have a very 'tight' design. The above covariance structure models are based on a simple precise design with simple precise questions to be answered. If the budding epidemiologist simply measures as many things as she can think of in a relatively unstructured way then the chances of successfully modelling these data in a way that can be replicated are pretty low. In practice most of the variables never get as far as the analysis; they are collected and forgotten. Instead of employing this 'shotgun' tactic, the following sequence should be followed:

1. What precise question (or possibly more than one, but not many) is the study being planned to answer?
2. How will that be formulated as a testable hypothesis within the context of a suitable statistical model (testing for group differences or non-zero regression coefficients in the presence of confounding variables, for example)?
3. What data (including multiple indicators of the key concepts) need to be collected to fit and estimate the parameters of a convincing model?
4. What is the most effective design and the required sample size?

When analysing the resulting data:

5. Sort out the correct measurement model prior to testing the substantive hypotheses.
6. Remember that association (correlation) does not imply causality.
7. Remember that there may be models other than the one you have fitted which describe the data equally well, and possibly even better.

The examples used so far in this text should go a long way to illustrate what is meant by points 1, 2, 3, 5, 6 and 7. Here, we deliberately do not go into problems of design, statistical power and sample size estimation. For many areas of statistical analysis they will be reasonably familiar. For a brief discussion of power calculations for covariance structure modelling we refer the reader to Dunn, Everitt and Pickles, 1993). One final point needs mentioning here. In this chapter all of the examples have been analysed assuming multivariate normality. This will often not be the case. Sometimes this can be solved using transformations of the measured variables. At other times it might be sensible to use methods of standard error estimation and significance testing that are *robust* to departures from normality (see, for example, Bentler, 1995, or Dunn, Everitt and Pickles, 1993, for further details). We will return briefly to this problem in the postscript at the end of Chapter 7.

6.7   Appendix 6

A   EQS program to fit a simple structural equation model to GHQ scores

```
/TITLE
 Structural Equation Model
 Data are GHQ scores from 12 students
 Odd vs Even subtotals on two occasions
/SPECIFICATION
 CASES=12;
 VARIABLES=4;
 METHOD=ML;
 MATRIX=CORRELATION;
 ANALYSIS=COVARIANCE;
/LABELS
 V1=ODD1;
 V2=EVEN1;
 V3=ODD2;
 V4=EVEN2;
 F1=DISTRESS1;
 F2=DISTRESS2;
/EQUATIONS
 V1=1*F1+E1;
 V2=1*F1+E2;
 V3=1*F2+E3;
 V4=1*F2+E4;
 F2=1*F1+D2;
/VARIANCES
 F1=1;
 D2=1*;
 E1 TO E4=1*;
/CONSTRAINTS
 (V1,F1)=(V2,F1)=(V3,F2)=(V4,F2);
 (E1,E1)=(E3,E3)=(E2,E2)=(E4,E4);
/MATRIX
 1.000
 0.8645 1.000
 0.9008 0.7516 1.000
 0.8597 0.8682 0.9075 1.000
/STANDARD DEVIATIONS
 3.5792 3.0189 3.0451 3.1909
/END
```

B   EQS program to fit a Wiley model to data on depression in children

```
/TITLE
 DEPRESSION IN CHILDREN - COLE ET AL, 1998
/SPECIFICATION
 CASES=330;
```

```
 VARIABLES=3;
 METHOD=ML;
 MATRIX=CORR;
 ANALYSIS=COV;
/LABELS
 V1=CDI1;  V2=CDI2;  V3=CDI3;
 F1=DEP1;  F2=DEP2;  F3=DEP3;
/EQUATIONS
 V1=F1+E1;
 V2=F2+E2;
 V3=F3+E3;
 F2=1*F1+D2;
 F3=1*F2+D3;
/VARIANCES
 F1=15*;
 E1 TO E3=10*;
 D2 TO D3=2*;
/CONSTRAINTS
 (E1,E1)=(E2,E2)=(E3,E3);
 (F2,F1)=(F3,F2);
 (D2,D2)=(D3,D3);
/MATRIX
 1.00
 0.72 1.00
 0.69 0.76 1.00
/STANDARD DEVIATIONS
 7.80 8.22 8.01
/END
```

C   EQS program to fit cross-lagged panel model for depression and anxiety

```
/TITLE
 ANXIETY & DEPRESSION IN CHILDREN - COLE ET AL, 1998
/SPECIFICATION
 CASES=330;
 VARIABLES=6;
 METHOD=ML;
 MATRIX=CORR;
 ANALYSIS=COV;
/LABELS
 V1=CDI1;  V2=RCMAS1;
 V3=CDI2;  V4=RCMAS2;
 V5=CDI3;  V6=RCMAS3;
 F1=DEP1;  F2=ANX1;
 F3=DEP2;  F4=ANX2;
 F5=DEP3;  F6=ANX3;
/EQUATIONS
 V1=F1+E1;
 V2=F2+E2;
```

```
 V3=F3+E3;
 V4=F4+E4;
 V5=F5+E5;
 V6=F6+E6;
 F3=1*F1+.1*F2+D3;
 F4=1*F1+.1*F2+D4;
 F5=1*F3+.1*F4+D5;
 F6=1*F3+.1*F4+D6;
/VARIANCES
 F1 TO F2=30*;
 E1 TO E6=10*;
 D3 TO D6=2*;
/COVARIANCES
 F1,F2=10*;
 E1,E2=1*; E3,E4=1*; E5,E6=1*;
/CONSTRAINTS
 (E1,E1)=(E3,E3)=(E5,E5);
 (E2,E2)=(E4,E4)=(E6,E6);
 (E1,E2)=(E3,E4)=(E5,E6);
 (F3,F1)=(F5,F3);
 (F3,F2)=(F5,F4);
 (F4,F1)=(F6,F3);
 (F4,F2)=(F6,F4);
 (D3,D3)=(D5,D5);
 (D4,D4)=(D6,D6);
/MATRIX
 1.00
 0.70 1.00
 0.72 0.58 1.00
 0.59 0.73 0.71 1.00
 0.69 0.57 0.76 0.66 1.00
 0.61 0.70 0.66 0.79 0.78 1.00
/STANDARD DEVIATIONS
 7.80 11.85 8.22 12.09 8.01 11.90
/END
```

D   EQS program to fit a two-group twin measurement model

```
/TITLE
 TWO GROUP TWIN MODEL - HEWITT ET AL, 1992 - MALE MZ TWINS
/SPECIFICATION
 CASES=96; VARIABLES=4; METHOD=ML;
 MATRIX=COV; ANALYSIS=COV; GROUPS=2;
/LABELS
 V1=MT1; V2=FT1;
 V3=MT2; V4=FT2;
 F1=PHE1; F2=PHE2;
/EQUATIONS
 V1=1*F1+E1;
```

```
 V2=1*F1+E2;
 V3=1*F2+E3;
 V4=1*F2+E4;
/VARIANCES
 F1 TO F2=1;
 E1 TO E4=1*;
/COVARIANCES
 F1,F2=0.5*;
 E1,E3=0.5*;
 E2,E4=0.5*;
/CONSTRAINTS
 (V1,F1)=(V3,F2);
 (V2,F1)=(V4,F2);
 (E1,E1)=(E3,E3);
 (E2,E2)=(E4,E4);
/MATRIX
 0.694
 0.312 0.638
 0.569 0.238 0.666
 0.308 0.461 0.293 0.647
/END
/TITLE
 TWO GROUP TWIN MODEL - HEWITT ET AL, 1992 - MALE DZ TWINS
/SPECIFICATION
 CASES=102; VARIABLES=4;
 METHOD=ML; MATRIX=COV; ANALYSIS=COV;
/LABELS
 V1=MT1; V2=FT1;
 V3=MT2; V4=FT2;
 F1=PHE1; F2=PHE2;
/EQUATIONS
 V1=1*F1+E1;
 V2=1*F1+E2;
 V3=1*F2+E3;
 V4=1*F2+E4;
/VARIANCES
 F1 TO F2=1;
 E1 TO E4=1*;
/COVARIANCES
 F1,F2=0.5*;
 E1,E3=0.5*;
 E2,E4=0.5*;
/CONSTRAINTS
 (1,V1,F1)=(2,V1,F1)=(2,V3,F2);
 (1,V2,F1)=(2,V2,F1)=(2,V4,F2);
 (1,E1,E1)=(2,E1,E1)=(2,E3,E3);
 (1,E2,E2)=(2,E2,E2)=(2,E4,E4);
 (1,E1,E3)=(2,E1,E3);
 (1,E2,E4)=(2,E2,E4);
```

```
/MATRIX
 0.565
 0.241 0.604
 0.291 0.137 0.488
 0.171 0.347 0.285 0.604
/END
```

E   EQS program to fit the ACE model for twin data with measurement errors

```
/TITLE
 TWO GROUP TWIN MODEL - HEWITT ET AL, 1992 - MALE MZ TWINS
/SPECIFICATION
 CASES=96; VARIABLES=4; METHOD=ML; MATRIX=COV; ANALYSIS=COV;
 GROUPS=2;
/LABELS
 V1=MT1; V2=FT1;
 V3=MT2; V4=FT2;
 F1=PHE1; F2=PHE2;
/EQUATIONS
 V1=F1+E1;
 V2=1*F1+E2;
 V3=F2+E3;
 V4=1*F2+E4;
 F1=1*F3+1*F4+D1;
 F2=1*F3+1*F4+D2;
/VARIANCES
 F3 TO F4=1;
 E1 TO E4=1*;
 D1 TO D2=1*;
/COVARIANCES
 E1,E3=0.5*;
 E2,E4=0.5*;
/CONSTRAINTS
 (V2,F1)=(V4,F2);  (E1,E1)=(E3,E3);
 (E2,E2)=(E4,E4);  (F1,F3)=(F2,F3);
 (F1,F4)=(F2,F4);  (D1,D1)=(D2,D2);
/INEQUALITIES
 (F1,F3)>0;        (F1,F4)>0;
/MATRIX
 0.694
 0.312 0.638
 0.569 0.238 0.666
 0.308 0.461 0.293 0.647
/END
/TITLE
 TWO GROUP TWIN MODEL - HEWITT ET AL, 1992 - MALE DZ TWINS
/SPECIFICATION
 CASES=102; VARIABLES=4; METHOD=ML; MATRIX=COV; ANALYSIS=COV;
/LABELS
```

```
 V1=MT1;  V2=FT1;
 V3=MT2;  V4=FT2;
 F1=PHE1;  F2=PHE2;
/EQUATIONS
 V1=F1+E1;
 V2=1*F1+E2;
 V3=F2+E3;
 V4=1*F2+E4;
 F1=1*F3+1*F4+D1;
 F2=1*F5+1*F4+D2;
/VARIANCES
 F3 TO F5=1;
 E1 TO E4=1*;
 D1 TO D2=1*;
/COVARIANCES
 E1,E3=0.5*;
 E2,E4=0.5*;
 F3,F5=0.5;
/CONSTRAINTS
 (1,V2,F1)=(2,V2,F1)=(2,V4,F2);
 (1,E1,E1)=(2,E1,E1)=(2,E3,E3);
 (1,E2,E2)=(2,E2,E2)=(2,E4,E4);
 (1,E1,E3)=(2,E1,E3);
 (1,E2,E4)=(2,E2,E4);
 (1,F1,F3)=(2,F1,F3)=(2,F2,F5);
 (1,F1,F4)=(2,F1,F4)=(2,F2,F4);
 (1,D1,D1)=(2,D1,D1)=(2,D2,D2);
/INEQUALITIES
 (F1,F3)>0;  (F1,F4)>0;  (F2,F5)>0;
/MATRIX
 0.565
 0.241 0.604
 0.291 0.137 0.488
 0.171 0.347 0.285 0.604
/END
```

7
Missing data

7.1 Introduction

Missing observations are characteristic of all psychiatric surveys and intervention studies. They may arise from the fact that particular measurements were not made on some individuals, or from the subsequent discovery that the measurements were either made or recorded in error and that they should therefore be dropped from the data set prior to any analysis. The fact that the measurements were never made might be accidental (i.e. *missing by happenstance*) or arise from a deliberate decision by the investigator (i.e. *missing by design*). Patients who have dropped out of a treatment trial provide an example of the former and two-phase epidemiological surveys provide an already familiar example of the latter. 'Accidentally missing' data can arise from a variety of reasons ranging, for example, from the administrative or technical incompetence of the investigator to the death or emigration of the subject. Perhaps the subject cannot be contacted at the time of a survey, or is too ill to participate in a diagnostic interview. Or perhaps the patient or informant simply refuses to take part in the investigation.

Traditionally investigators have coped with missing value problems in multivariate data sets by analysing only that part of the data with no missing observations (*complete-case analysis*). Although in some situations this strategy might be warranted, in general the data analysis should use all available information. The complete-case analysis is likely to be inefficient (unless the number of subjects with missing data is relatively small) but, more importantly, it might lead to biased estimates due to the fact that the complete cases are not representative of the sample as a whole. We have already come across these potential biases in discussing strategies for dealing with two-phase studies of instrument validity (Chapter 3) and illness prevalence (Chapter 5). In longitudinal cohort studies the subjects who drop out, or who are otherwise lost to follow-up, will differ systematically from those who remain in the study (see, for example, Gornbein *et al.*, 1992). Table 7.1 (from Diggle, 1998) gives the reported reasons for dropout from a randomised controlled trial of the effects

Table 7.1   Frequency distribution of reasons for dropout from a drug trial for the treatment of chronic schizophrenia (number recruited = 523) (from Diggle, 1998)

Abnormal lab result	4
Adverse experience	26
Inadequate response	183
Intercurrent illness	3
Lost to follow-up	3
Other reason	7
Unco-operative	25
Withdrew consent	19

of risperidone, haloperidol or a placebo in the treatment of chronic schizophrenia. There were 523 patients who agreed to be randomised in this trial. Clearly, adverse experiences, inadequate responses, withdrawal of consent, and so on, are unlikely to be completely random. They are likely to be related to the allocated treatment, for example.

In Chapter 3 we discussed so-called verification biases arising from the failure (either accidental or otherwise) to validate all screening data with a diagnostic interview. In earlier chapters (particularly Chapters 3 and 5) we have also dealt with missing data patterns that have arisen by design (i.e. two-phase or double sampling). Another example is the balanced incomplete blocks design (BIBD) for a reliability study (see Sections 2.7 and 7.5). In the present chapter we discuss missing data in a bit more detail and, in particular, pursue the use of multiple-group covariance structure modelling as a strategy for dealing with missing quantitative data in studies involving multiple indicators. First, however, we briefly describe the possible patterns of missing data (Section 7.2) and missing data mechanisms (Section 7.3).

7.2   Patterns of missing data

Brick and Kalton (1996) describe four sources of missing data. *Total* or *unit non-response* is probably the most familiar. Here the patient or informant provides no information at all. Data on this subject are completely missing. Either the subject is unavailable for interview, for example, or cannot be traced, or refuses to take part in the investigation. This description, however, is slightly misleading since we usually know the identity of the missing individual and often have some demographic information such as their age and sex. Compensation for total non-response is usually made by *weighting adjustments* in which the respondents (i.e. those who provide the required information) are assigned greater weight in the analysis in order to represent the non-respondents. The use of these weighting adjustments is very similar to the way in which it was described in Chapters 2 and 3. The second source of missing data (particularly with respect to epidemiological surveys) is *incomplete coverage* arising from the inadequacy of the survey's sampling frame. Here there are patients or informants who have no chance of selection for interview, say, simply because they are not listed on the sampling frame. Again, compensation is usually made through the use of weights, but here the weights have to be determined by reference to external data sources (by comparing the demographic structure of the *sampled population* (via the sampling frame) with the demographic structure of the intended *target population* as determined by a national census, for example). In the case of total non-response, however, weights can be determined by comparing the structure of the actual sample with that of the sampled population.

A third source of missing data is *item non-response* in which there may be one or more variables for which there is inadequate information provided by the respondent. The pattern of missing data might also vary from one respondent to another. Item non-response can arise from a variety of reasons. A patient or informant may refuse to answer a particular question, or may not understand what the question means, or simply not know the answer. The interviewer may forget to ask the question or forget to record the answer. The answer may be coded incorrectly, and so on. The most frequent form of compensation for item non-response is *imputation* (assigning a value to the missing response). Finally, Brick and Kalton (1996) discuss *partial non-response*. Partial non-response involves a substantial number of item non-responses, but typically they are not occurring in a haphazard way. In a two-phase prevalence survey, for example, all subjects (the first-phase sample) might provide demographic information together with the results from the screening questionnaire – but only selected sub-samples (the second-phase respondents) are given the structured or semi-structured psychiatric interview. If the second-phase respondents provide a single measurement (psychiatric diagnosis, for example) then this is an example of item non-response. If, however, they provide, say, a detailed breakdown of their symptoms together with further background information, then this is clearly an example of partial non-response. Compensation for partial non-response can be handled by using either weighting or imputation.

Another familiar pattern of partial non-responses arises from dropout in a longitudinal cohort or panel study. Typically we would start with, say, a sample (panel) of m subjects and aim to assess them on each of a number of distinct occasions (waves). Once someone drops out of the study, then it is usually the case that they are lost and do not provide any information at any subsequent occasions. A subject, for example, may withdraw after the second wave of a planned six-wave panel study. That person will have observations for waves one and two, but missing data for waves three to six. There will, of course, be distinct patterns of partial response dependent on the timing of the dropout.

7.3   Missing data mechanisms

In compensating for missing values it is vital that we bear in mind our explicit or implicit assumptions concerning the way the missing data have arisen. Using the terminology of Little and Rubin (1987), the simplest assumption is that the missing observations are *missing completely at random* (*MCAR*), that is, there is no information that we have collected, or might have collected, that would enable us to predict who might have missing information. In other words, MCAR refers to the situation where the probability that a particular observation is missing does not depend upon either its own value (had it been observed) or the value of any other observation. For data *missing at random* (*MAR*) the probability of an observation being missing may depend upon the values of other observed measures but not upon those that have not been observed. Consider, for example, a two-phase survey to validate a screening questionnaire. All first-phase respondents provide fallible screening information. Only a sub-sample of these is given the validation interview. If the second-phase sample were to be chosen without reference to the screening (or any other) information, then the validation data would be MCAR. An alternative strategy (the one used in Chapter 3) is to interview a high proportion of the screen-positives (often all of them) but only a small sub-sample (say 20%) of the screen-negatives. Providing the sampling mechanism is completely random within the strata determined by the screen outcome, then this produces validation data that are MAR. If the probability of a missing validation interview is dependent on the subject's true psychiatric status, even after conditioning on the screen outcome and other information, then the missing data mechanism is referred to as being *informative* or *non-ignorable* (Little and Rubin, 1987). In addition to any second-phase sampling fractions determined by the investigator, the probability of a selected second-phase subject agreeing to be interviewed is likely be influenced by the severity and other characteristics of their illness. The concept of ignorability as discussed by Little and Rubin is a difficult one but can be interpreted as any statistical mechanism for generating missing observations that is **neither MCAR nor** MAR.

Most of the methods discussed in the following sections (weighting and imputation, for example) are justified by the assumption that the missing data mechanism is not informative (ignorable). That is, we assume that the missing data are either MCAR or MAR. When the only missing data have arisen by design then, of course, we know whether our assumptions are justified. The BIBD for an inter-rater reliability study, for example, produces data that are MCAR. Two-phase epidemiological survey data usually generate second-phase data that are MAR. In both cases, however, we are assuming that all the selected subjects are complying with the request to provide the required information. If not, then the MCAR or MAR assumptions might be challenged. Often, however, we have to take these assumptions on trust. This is not always the case, however, and Diggle (1998), for example, provides a good discussion of modelling dropout mechanisms in the analysis of longitudinal data.

7.4   Weighting and imputation

By now the use of adjustment weights should be reasonably familiar. We will briefly recap using the two-phase survey data from Cantabria (Chapter 5). In the first phase the respondents were screened for signs of psychological distress (using the GP's assessment and the GHQ). Of the 514 screen-negatives, 42 were sub-sampled for the second-phase interview. The sampling fraction was $42/514$ and the corresponding probability weight was therefore $514/42 = 12.238$. Of the 309 screen-positives, 161 were interviewed in the second phase. Here the sampling fraction was $161/309$ and the corresponding probability weight was $309/161 = 1.919$. When calculated separately for the two sexes, the probability weights for men were 12.611 and 2.366 for screen-negatives and screen-positives, respectively. The corresponding weights for women were 11.958 and 1.767 (see Pickles *et al.*, 1995).

Imputation methods come in a variety of forms. Essentially, imputation involves filling the gap (the missing observation) with an estimate based on a knowledge of the variables that have been observed. The simplest is possibly the average for that variable calculated from information provided by non-missing respondents. A better approach is to use the average from a similar stratum of the non-missing respondents. We also might use information from correlated variables to construct a regression equation to predict the value for the missing data item. Consider the particularly simple situation from a two-phase survey where the only information available is the subject's screen status (probable case or probable non-case) together with their sex. We wish to impute the result of a missing diagnostic interview (case or non-case). Here we would like to impute missing interview outcomes for four possible classes of subject (screen status crossed by sex) – the four *imputation classes*. One can replace the missing responses by the proportion of cases (as determined by interview) amongst the subjects with non-missing data in the appropriate imputation class. For example, the proportion of cases in the second-phase screen-positive men in the Spanish survey was $22/41 = 0.537$. We can replace the missing values for caseness in those first-phase screen-positive men who were not interviewed by the value 0.537, and similarly for the other imputation classes, and then proceed with the analysis as if we had no missing values (we would have to be careful in the way we might proceed with the analysis, however, as 0.537 is no longer an example of a binary response!). This *deterministic* imputation would yield unbiased estimates and is, in fact, equivalent to the above method of probability weighting. A subtle variation on this theme is a form of *stochastic* imputation: to randomly select the value of 1 for the missing observation (1 = case) with a probability of 0.537 (and similarly using the other three imputation classes) and again estimate the overall prevalence of cases. This is an example of what is known as hot-deck imputation (Brick and Kalton, 1996). Reilly and Pepe (1997) discuss the similarities of hot-deck imputation and weighted estimation. We will not go into any further detail here.

NB Just in case the reader may not have noticed, great care should be made in the use of either weights or imputation to avoid being lulled into thinking that we now have a full data set. The use of weights or imputation (or any other statistical device, for that matter) does not create data! You do not get something for nothing. Dunn *et al.* (1999) illustrate how the use of weighting adjustments, for example, with inappropriate software might lead one seriously astray. Whether the data set appears to be complete (after imputation) or has been expanded to be in some way representative of what might have been collected (after weighting adjustments), it is vital that we make sure that we calculate appropriate standard errors, confidence intervals and *P*-values using methodology that explicitly recognises the true state of affairs.

7.5   Data missing by design

Consider a relatively simple measurement problem. We wish to calibrate one measurement method against another when it is possible to use one or other of them on an individual subject or specimen, but not both. Consider, for example, a hypothetical set of measurements made in a clinical laboratory. There are four measurements available: A, B, C and D. The first two, A and B, do not involve destruction of all of the material under test and can be made on the same specimens of material. The second two, C and D, both involve destruction of the specimen and each require most of the available material to be used in the assay. A particular specimen can yield either C or D, but not both. A simple design for a method comparison study might involve getting measurements A and B on all specimens and then **randomly** allocating specimens to be processed to give either C or D. This design would yield two groups of specimens – both with data that are MCAR – one having measurements on A, B and C and the other with A, B and D. By fitting a factor model simultaneously to these two groups the relative calibration of C and D can be undertaken, even though both C and D are never available for the same specimen. In each case we assume a single common factor model and all parameters describing the distribution of A and B (together with the common factor) are constrained to be the same in the two groups. Those for C and D are left free to be estimated but can then be constrained to be equal by across-group constraints to test whether the two methods have the same characteristics. It is relatively straightforward to think of an analogous situation in psychiatric epidemiology. A and B, for example, might be simple screening questionnaires. C and D could be alternative interviewers or structured psychiatric interviews. It is more difficult in this context to convince oneself that there is no contamination (correlated errors) between measures – see Lewis *et al.*, 1992, for example – but even so the design has certain advantages. It is a design that is applied to a completely different substantive problem (compliance–response relationships) in Section 7.6 and we leave a detailed discussion of the analysis strategy until then. The multiple-group factor analysis approach (with appropriate constraints across groups) can also be applied to means/covariance data arising from a BIBD inter-rater reliability study (see Section 2.5). Dunn (1989, pp. 101–105) gives a detailed description of how this is done and, again, we will not concentrate on the practicalities here.

Before we move on to further designs and models for covariance structures with missing data, let us look at a very simple type of intervention study. Suppose we have a group of patients who might benefit from a new form of psychotherapy, counselling or case management. And suppose, for example, we randomly allocate these patients to two management strategies. One group is offered 'treatment as usual' and the other 'treatment as usual' plus a referral or attachment to a new counsellor or case manager. In a conventional design for this study we would seek informed consent prior to randomisation, but several investigators might advocate the use of a form of the *randomised consent design* (Zelen, 1979). According to this design the patients would first be randomised and consent would only be sought from those offered the novel treatment or management. Consent would not be sought from the 'treatment as usual' group or, at most, consent might be sought to collect outcome data on them. For our purposes it does not matter whether the conventional RCT design or the Zelen design is actually used. We then observe a simple binary outcome: has the patient got better (yes/no)?

Assume that we have the outcome on all patients (i.e. no outcome data are missing). To test the effect of allocation to counselling we simply carry out an *intention-to-treat* analysis by estimating the proportion of patients who recover in each treatment group, whether or not they took up the offer of counselling. Knowing that some of the patients who were offered counselling did not take up the offer, we might also ask: what was the effect on outcome of actually receiving counselling? In other words, what was the impact of patient compliance? Clearly we do not have any compliance data on the patients who received 'treatment as usual' but let us assume that we have compliance data (yes/no) on all those offered counselling. The compliance data are MCAR by design (randomised allocation to the two groups).

An approach to the latter question was suggested by Sommer and Zeger (1991) and their work has been extended by Cuzick, Edwards and Segnan (1997) to model the joint effects of non-compliance and contamination in clinical trials. Sommer and Zeger assumed that, as a direct result of randomisation, the proportion of the compliers in the two arms of the trial is the same. We do not have information on this for the 'treatment as usual' group because they do not have anything to comply with. We therefore estimate the common proportion from that observed in the group offered counselling. The second assumption was that the recovery rate was the same in non-compliers, irrespective of whether they were actually offered counselling. These two assumptions, and how they lead to an estimate of the treatment difference for the compliant patient group, are illustrated by reference to Table 7.2.

In the group of 100 patients offered counselling, 70 took up the offer. Of these, 55 improved. Thirty patients did not take up the offer of counselling and only five of these improved. In the 'treatment as usual' group we can estimate that 30 of them would not have taken up the offer of counselling if they had been offered it (that is, we assume that the rates would be the same in each group). Of these we can estimate that five would have got better. All

Table 7.2 A hypothetical trial of counselling: observed counts

Group 1 Counselling ($N = 100$)	
Number compliers $= 70$; number of these improved $= 55$	
Non-compliers $= 30$; number these improved	$= 5$
Overall improvement rate	$= 60/100$
Proportion improved in non-compliant group	$= 5/30$
Proportion improved in compliant group	$= 55/70$
Group 2 'Treatment as usual' ($N = 100$)	
Number improved $= 30$	
Estimated number of non-compliers	$= 30$ (from above)
Estimated number of improved non-compliers	$= 5$ (from above)
Estimated number of potential compliers	$= 70$ (from above)
Estimated number of improved potential compliers	$= 30 - 5$
	$= 25$
Overall improvement rate	$= 30/100$
Improvement rate for compliant group	$= 25/70$
Estimated group differences	
As allocated (intention-to-treat)	$= 60/100 - 30/100$
	$= 0.30$
In potential compliers	$= 55/70 - 25/70$
	$= 30/70$
	$= 0.43$

we actually observe in the 'treatment as usual' group, however, is that there were 30 improvements out of a total of 100. But we can estimate that the number of potentially compliant patients would have been 70 (i.e. the same as in the group offered counselling) and that, of these, 25 (i.e. 30 − 5) have got better. We compare the improvement rate in those that took up counselling (55/70) with that in those who would have taken up counselling had they been offered it (25/70). The difference is 30/70 (i.e. 0.43). The conventional intention-to-treat analysis would have compared 60/100 with 30/100 (i.e. a difference of 0.30). We do not wish to go into any further details here concerning the precision of these estimates but refer the reader to Cuzich *et al.* (1998) for further discussion. The main point of introducing this example was so that it could act as a starting point (together with the earlier part of this section on multiple-group factor analysis) for the application of a similar logic to covariance structure modelling of randomised trials in which compliance has been measured.

7.6 Modelling compliance–response relationships in clinical trials

Here we discuss how we might model a quantitative response as a function of two or more quantitative measures of compliance. We stress that the models considered here may not be appropriate for a given clinical trial, but use simulated data to illustrate how we might deal with missing data in the context of a randomised intervention study (see Dunn, 1999, for further details). The missing data are assumed to be missing by design (in this case, being MCAR).

Recent methodological work on statistical modelling of the effect of compliance in randomised clinical trials takes as its starting point the seminal paper of Efron and Feldman (1991). These authors investigate the recovery of true dose–response curves from the treatment and control compliance–response curves. They treat compliance as an inherent characteristic of a patient that is not influenced by the outcome of the allocation of the patient to the treatment or the control group. In their commentary on Efron and Feldman's paper, Zeger and Liang (1991) develop the former authors' ideas but focus on the situation where compliance data from the two groups are not comparable, either because a placebo could not be used in the control group or because the placebo–compliance pattern was thought to be irrelevant. Zeger and Liang demonstrate that it is possible to estimate the required dose–response curve on the assumption that: (1) the treatment, if administered, would have a similar effect regardless of a patient's propensity to comply and (2) the compliance–response function is linear. The slope of the compliance–response function is easily estimated using linear regression for the treatment group patients, and that for the controls is then inferred by further assuming (a) that the response at zero compliance (i.e. the intercept term) is the same for treatment and control groups and (b) that randomisation ensures that the distribution of the propensity to comply to treatment is the same in the two groups. The estimated slope for the controls is obtained by simply dividing the difference between mean response in the control group and the common intercept by the mean compliance in the treatment group.

The problem is considered here as one of exposure measurement, with true exposure to the therapeutic drug, for example, being regarded as a hidden or latent variable. Exposure is measured by two types of manifest or observed variable: (a) indicators of compliance such as pills taken or concentrations of drug metabolites or other bio-markers in blood or urine, and (b) the observed effects of exposure (i.e. response to treatment). Note that the precise meaning of the word 'exposure' is dependent on context – obviously in a placebo-controlled drug trial the placebo-treated controls never get exposed to the active drug. 'Exposure' here could be thought of as an error-free measure of propensity to comply. In other contexts (psychotherapy, for example) it might be a measure of belief, motivation or propensity to participate or engage in therapy. Note also that both compliance and response measures might be considered as outcome variables – they are both 'effects' of the hidden exposure. Here, in order to simplify the discussion we will assume that all outcome measures are conditionally independent given true exposure. Assuming that both compliance and response measurements are quantitative, and that each measurement has a simple linear relationship with true exposure, we have the following:

$$V_j = \alpha_j + \beta_j F_1 + E_j \tag{7.1}$$

where F_1 is the subject's unknown true exposure and V_j is the jth measurement of outcome made on the subject. Note that, for the present, in the use of the Vs as outcomes we are not distinguishing observed measures of compliance from treatment responses. The factor, F_1, and the E_js are uncorrelated random variables with expected values of μ and 0, respectively. Let the variance of F_1 be σ^2 and that of E_j be σ_j^2. The parameters of the model are μ and the α_j and β_j, together with the variances, σ^2 and σ_j^2. The model represented in (7.1) is mathematically equivalent to the familiar factor analysis model with the familiar structure for the expected covariance matrix of the Vs. Here we are also interested in estimating intercept terms, so we also note that

$$E(V_j) = \mu_j = \alpha_j + \beta_j \mu \tag{7.2}$$

For identifiability (setting the scale of measurement) we constrain $\alpha_1 = 0$ and $\beta_1 = 1$. Again, we know that all other parameters are estimable (i.e. the model is identified) as long as we have three or more manifest indicators (the V_js). In the present context this implies either (a) at least one response measurement and at least two compliance measures, or (b) at least two response measurements and at least one compliance indicator. The model is fitted by comparing the predicted covariance matrix together with the expected values of the means, μ_j, with their observed counterparts from the sample. Here we assume multivariate normality and fit by maximum likelihood.

The model in (7.1) is illustrated graphically in Figure 7.1. Cox and Wermuth (1996) discuss the use of factor analysis models in the context of predicting a response from a set of error-prone explanatory variables and an alternative graphical representation is provided by Figure 8.1 of their book. Both graphical representations emphasise that **observed** indicators of compliance are effects of the latent variable. They can be thought of as intermediate outcomes rather than explanatory variables. The main response is also an effect of the hidden variable and here it is considered to be conditionally independent of

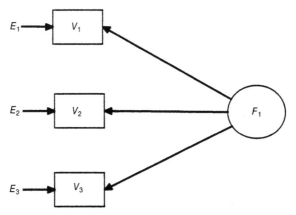

Figure 7.1   Path diagram illustrating compliance–response relationships.
Key:
F_1 – the single common factor (compliance, C)
V_1 – first measurement of compliance (X_1)
V_2 – second measurement of compliance (X_2)
V_3 – response (Y)
E_1, E_2 and E_3 – residuals associated with V_1, V_2 and V_3, respectively (note that E_1 and E_2 are interpreted as measurement errors whilst E_3 is a random disturbance term that is not necessarily a measurement error).

measured compliance measures, given the value of the hidden variable. There is no direct path in these graphs between observed compliance and outcome. Figure 7.1 looks superficially like a simple measurement model. This is not the case, however. As an aid to correct interpretation the labelling of the variables has been changed. The latent variable (F_1) is a measure of true compliance (C). The variables X_1 and X_2 are observed (manifest) measures of compliance (corresponding to V_1 and V_2, above). The corresponding measurement errors are E_1 and E_2. That part of the path diagram which includes C, X_1, X_2, E_1 and E_2 constitutes the measurement model. The construct equation simply links true compliance (C) with observed response (Y). Y is equivalent to V_3, above, and D (E_3) is the random deviation of the predicted response from that actually observed. It is not a measurement error.

Returning to the context of a clinical trial, we will assume that we have two randomly allocated groups of subjects: treated and controls. These groups will provide means and covariance matrices for the response(s) and compliance measures. It may be the case, however, that one or more of the compliance measures may not be available for anyone in the control group. Note that if the only factor which determines whether these compliance measures are available is, in fact, treatment allocation (i.e. randomisation) then this gives rise to data that are MCAR. We fit a factor analysis model to each of the group's summary statistics (means, variances and covariances) simultaneously. We constrain the parameters describing the behaviour of the compliance measures with respect to true exposure (i.e. the parameters of the measurement model) to be equal across the groups – whether or not the measures are available for both groups or available for the treatment group only. We may also constrain the mean and variance of true exposure to be the same for the two groups – testing whether compliance itself is dependent upon group membership.

As for the response(s), we constrain the intercept terms (the αs) for a given response to be the same for the treatment and control groups – that is, the response in both groups is assumed to be the same when there is zero exposure (Zeger and Liang, 1991). Finally, we leave the regression coefficients (the βs) for the response variables (Y) to be separately estimated for the two groups. These measure the 'causal effects' of exposure to treatment and, if the treatment is effective, we would expect them to differ for treated and control groups. The compliance–response curve in the treatment group can be compared with that in the control group, even though an individual patient cannot be simultaneously exposed to both experimental conditions.

Simple linear regression is a special case of fitting model (7.1) where we have a single response and a single error-free measure of compliance/exposure (here the error term is dropped from the model, or, alternatively, its variance is constrained to be 0). ANCOVA – fitting regressions to the two groups of subjects (with or without constraints) – is straightforward in EQS, as is the estimation suggested by Zeger and Liang (1991) for the case when either we do not have compliance measured in the control group, or we wish to ignore it. For the Zeger and Liang approach we have to constrain the mean and variance of the true exposure to be the same in both groups. From there we can return to the basic regression models but use a vector of fallible indicators of compliance rather than a single measure that is assumed to be error-free. Alternatively, we can stick with the Zeger and Liang approach (that is, ignoring compliance data for the controls) and again move to a more realistic measurement model for the treatment group measures. An example of an EQS program to fit the Zeger and Liang model is given in Appendix 7.

To illustrate our ideas we have simulated data for 1000 subjects according to the following model:

$$V_1(= F_1) = \mu + \delta_1 \qquad \text{(true exposure)}$$

$$V_2 \qquad = F_1 + \varepsilon_2 \qquad \text{(fallible indicator of compliance} - X_1)$$

$$V_3 \qquad = F_1 + \varepsilon_3 \qquad \text{(fallible indicator of compliance} - X_2)$$

$$V_4 \qquad = \alpha_4 + \beta_4 F_1 + \varepsilon_4 \quad \text{(response} - Y)$$

where $\mu = 70$ and $\alpha_4 = 50$. $\beta_4 = 4$ for 'treated' subjects ($N = 498$) and $\beta_4 = 1$ for controls ($N = 502$). Allocation to treatment or control groups was determined at random.

The random variables δ_1, ε_2, ε_3 and ε_4 were all Gaussian variates with zero mean and standard deviations of 15, 12, 15 and 15, respectively (note that the choice of these standard errors is completely arbitrary but the resulting reliabilities might be thought to be reasonably realistic). The reliabilities of V_2 and V_3 were, therefore, 0.613 (i.e. $\text{Var}(\delta_1)/\text{Var}(\delta_1 + \varepsilon_2)$) and 0.500 (i.e. $\text{Var}(\delta_1)/\text{Var}(\delta_1 + \varepsilon_3)$), respectively. Summary statistics for the two groups are shown in Table 7.3.

Table 7.3 Summary statistics for simulated compliance–response data set ($N = 1000$)

Group 1 (Treatment)
$N = 498$

	V_1	V_2	V_3	V_4
Mean	69.7247	70.0916	69.2183	327.5066
Standard deviation	14.2918	18.9657	21.0800	59.9957

Correlation/Covariance
(below/above diagonal, respectively)

	V_1	V_2	V_3	V_4
V_1	–	202.8679	214.2850	832.5316
V_2	0.7484	–	210.1197	851.3152
V_3	0.7113	0.5256	–	872.5090
V_4	0.9709	0.7482	0.6899	–

Group 2 (Control)
$N = 502$

	V_1	V_2	V_3	V_4
Mean	70.6935	70.5985	72.0170	121.0688
Standard deviation	14.8374	19.0190	21.8193	20.4429

Correlation/Covariance
(below/above diagonal, respectively)

	V_1	V_2	V_3	V_4
V_1	–	225.5492	233.3267	212.1016
V_2	0.7993	–	234.3393	227.1442
V_3	0.7207	0.5647	–	236.5372
V_4	0.6993	0.5842	0.5303	–

We start by simultaneously fitting a simple factor model to moments matrices (means, variances and covariances) from both groups. Each factor model is for three manifest variables – two fallible indicators of compliance (V_2 and V_3) and the response (V_4). All parameters involving the fallible indicators are constrained to be common to both groups, as is the intercept term for the response (α_4). Although there is no necessity to introduce constraints on the factor (F_1 – the true exposure) we have actually constrained both the mean and the variance to be common to both groups. The only parameters free to have separate estimates in the two groups are, in fact, β_4 and the variance of the residuals for the response (that is the variance of ε_4). Model identifiability is achieved by setting the intercept term and regression coefficient for V_2 (that is α_2 and β_2) to be 0 and 1, respectively.

Fitting the model using maximum likelihood produces a chi-square of 6.54 with seven degrees of freedom. The estimates of β_4 in the treatment and control groups are 4.010 (s.e. 0.071) and 1.037 (s.e. 0.066), respectively.

In a drug trial we might have access to two indicators of compliance – some sort of pill count, for example, and a metabolite measurement (see, for example, Urquhart and De Klerk, 1998). Both measures will be available for members of the treatment group but, clearly, the metabolite measure cannot be available in the case of those receiving a placebo (although it would be possible to put an inert marker into a placebo for monitoring purposes). Assume that V_2 is a metabolite measurement that is not available in our control group. V_3, a pill count, is available for both groups. We simply drop any reference to V_2 in the control group and re-fit the above confirmatory factor analysis model – again simultaneously fitting the same model to both groups, together with the relevant constraints. The resulting chi-square is 5.314 with three degrees of freedom. The estimates of β_4 are 4.014 (s.e. 0.108) and 1.046 (s.e. 0.104) for the treatment and control groups, respectively.

Consider the situation where we have two (or more) compliance measures available for the treatment group, but none for the controls. Again, we acknowledge that our compliance indicators are not error-free. We can extend the Zeger and Liang approach by simply dropping V_3 from the control group in the previous model. The required EQS program is provided in Appendix 7. In summary, we are (1) allowing for the error in the compliance measures by modelling their effect through a confirmatory factor analysis model, and (2) imposing the Zeger and Liang assumptions on the effects and distribution of a latent variable (F_1) rather than any of the compliance measures themselves. The model is only just identified and so we cannot use a chi-square to test its fit. The required estimates for β_4 are 4.152 (s.e. 0.235) and 1.207 (0.237).

7.7   Postscript

So much for missing values. Let us now try to summarise the main thrust of this text. I have tried to cover material that appears to give psychiatric epidemiology a unique flavour. I have put a lot of stress on measurement error models and, in fact, might be accused of giving too much space to factor analytic and other co-variance structure models. Indeed, many mathematical statisticians might say that I should not have given these two methodologies any space at all! By setting aside a complete chapter on missing data and also by giving a fair amount of space to two-phase sampling methodologies, I have also given a lot of importance to questions concerning what to do about missing observations. One other area, which has not received as much attention as it perhaps deserved, is the question of non-normality. Many distributions in psychiatry are distinctly non-Gaussian. The reverse J-shape of psychological distress or depression scores obtained from community survey samples is one well-known example. Categorising subjects into so-called cases and non-cases, of course, gets around some of these problems, and much of the material for binary responses in multiphase sampling is not dependent on the frequency distributions of the screening questionnaire scores. On the whole, covariance structure software such as EQS is likely to produce reasonable parameter estimates through the use of so-called maximum likelihood fitting algorithms (they are only maximum likelihood if the data are truly multivariate normal) and the choice of fitting algorithm rarely makes too much difference to the value of the estimates. They are asymptotically consistent (see Bollen, 1989, for example). Standard error estimation and significance testing, however, are likely to be more of a problem. Most software packages for covariance structure modelling contain procedures for the robust estimation of standard errors and increasingly they are likely also to contain bootstrap, jackknife and Monte Carlo simulation facilities. It is also possible to transform the original measurements to normality and this is often successful. It might not, however, be a particularly appropriate approach when we are jointly modelling mean and covariance structures. We might also group the data into broad intervals and generate *polychoric correlations* (also used for ordinal variables), for example. There are lots of things one might try and I will simply warn readers that they need to be careful. Try to look at data sets from as many angles as possible. Do not naively and mechanically fit any model to a set of data – there are pitfalls for the unwary everywhere! Do not assume that the distributional assumptions can be ignored or taken for granted.

Finally, I need to mention software. Virtually all of the data analyses described in this text have been carried out using two packages: *Stata* (for binary data, particularly involving the use of probability or expansion weights) and EQS (for single and multigroup covariance structure models). The choice is entirely a personal one and there are many other high-quality commercial packages that will be able to do the job equally well. This applies particularly to software for covariance structure modelling. I have included listings for many of the EQS jobs and *Stata* commands, not necessarily to imply that EQS or *Stata* is the software one should use, but mainly to illustrate **precisely** how I have fitted the models. Readers can check every line of my programs and, where appropriate, replicate my approach using other software packages. It will also enable them to check whether I have made any mistakes! One thing that I cannot stress too much, however, is that when using weighted logistic regression algorithms users of software must ensure that the standard error estimates are correctly calculated. Here we are concerned with the correct use of probability, expansion or sampling weights (all terms having essentially the same meaning). We are not concerned with frequency weights (this is where we appear to start getting something for nothing – have another look at the last paragraph of Section 7.4). When reading software manuals concerning weighted algorithms first check whether they distinguish the various types (*Stata*, for example, deals with weights that are described under several headings: 'frequency', 'probability', 'analytic' or 'importance'). If the software only mentions one type of weight then it is important that the potential user of the software understands fully what the word 'weight' means and its implications for a given approach to analysis.

7.8   Appendix 7: EQS program to fit a compliance–response model

```
/TITLE
 Two-Group Compliance Model - TREATMENT GROUP
 SECOND DATASET
/SPECIFICATION
 CASES=498;
 VARIABLES=4;
 METHOD=ML;
 MATRIX=CORRELATION;
 ANALYSIS=MOMENT;
 GROUPS=2;
```

```
/LABELS
 V1=COMP1;
 V2=COMP2;
 V3=COMP3;
 V4=RESPONSE;
 F1=TCOMP;
/EQUATIONS                      ! /EQUATIONS
 V1=F1;                         !  V2=F1+E2;
 V4=50*V999+4*F1+E4;            !  V3=1*V999+1*F1+E3;
 F1=70*V999+D1;                 !  V4=50*V999+4*F1+E4;
/VARIANCES                      !  F1=70*V999+D1;
 D1=225*;                       ! /VARIANCES
 E4=225*;                       !  D1=225*; E2=144*; E3=225*; E4=225*;
/MATRIX
 1.000
 0.7484  1.000
 0.7113  0.5256  1.000
 0.9709  0.7482  0.6899  1.000
/MEANS
 69.7247  70.0916  69.2183  327.5066
/STANDARD DEVIATIONS
 14.2918  18.9657  21.0800  59.9957
/END
/TITLE
 Two-Group Compliance Model - CONTROL GROUP
/SPECIFICATION
 CASES=502;
 VARIABLES=4;
 METHOD=ML;
 MATRIX=CORRELATION;
 ANALYSIS=MOMENT;
/LABELS
 V1=COMP1;
 V2=COMP2;
 V3=COMP3;
 V4=RESPONSE;
 F1=TCOMP;
/EQUATIONS
 V4=50*V999+1*F1+E4;
 F1=70*V999+D1;
/VARIANCES
 D1=225*;
 E4=225*;
/CONSTRAINTS
 (1,D1,D1)=(2,D1,D1);
 (1,V4,V999)=(2,V4,V999);
 (1,F1,V999)=(2,F1,V999);
/MATRIX
 1.000
```

```
 0.7993   1.000
 0.7207   0.5647   1.000
 0.6993   0.5842   0.5303   1.000
/MEANS
 70.6935   70.5985   72.0170   121.0688
/STANDARD DEVIATIONS
 14.8374   19.0190   21.8193   20.4429
/END
```

* The commands indicated to the right of the ! signs would convert this program into one for fitting the more realistic model, which allows for measurement error. '!' is a comment symbol in EQS and anything to the right of '!' is ignored. The program lines for the control group remain the same in both analyses.

References

Agresti, A. (1992). Modelling patterns of agreement and disagreement. *Statistical Methods in Medical Research* **1**, 201–218.

Amador, X.F., Strauss, D.H., Yale, S.A. *et al.* (1993). Assessment of insight in psychosis. *American Journal of Psychiatry* **150**, 873–879.

American Psychiatric Association (1987). *Diagnostic and Statistical Manual of Mental Disorders* (3rd edition revised) (DSM-IIIR). Washington, DC: APA.

Andreasen, N.C. (1982). Negative symptoms in schizophrenia. Definition and reliability. *Archives of General Psychiatry* **39**, 784–788.

Andreasen, N.C. (1983). *The Scale for the Assessment of Negative Symptoms (SANS)*. Iowa City: University of Iowa.

Andreasen, N.C. (1984). *The Scale for the Assessment of Positive Symptoms (SAPS)*. Iowa City: University of Iowa.

Bartholomew, D.J. (1987). *Latent Variable Models and Factor Analysis*. London: Griffin.

Bartholomew, D.J. (1996). *The Statistical Approach to Social Measurement*. San Diego, CA: Academic Press.

Bech, P. (1981). Rating scales for affective disorder: their validity and consistency. *Acta Psychiatrica Scandinavica*, Supplement **295**.

Beck, A.T. and Beamesderfer, A. (1974). Assessment of depression: the depression inventory. In *Psychological Measurements in Psychopharmacology* (P. Pichot, ed.), Vol. 7, pp. 151–169. Paris: Kargel-Basel.

Beck, A.T., Ward, C.H., Mendelson, M. *et al.* (1961). An inventory for measuring depression. *Archives of General Psychiatry* **4**, 561–571.

Beck, A.T., Wiseman, A.W., Lester, D. *et al.* (1974). The assessment of pessimism: the Hopelessness Scale. *Journal of Consulting and Clinical Psychology* **42**, 861–865.

Beck, A.T., Epstein, N., Brown, G. *et al.* (1988). An inventory for measuring anxiety: psychometric properties. *Journal of Consulting and Clinical Psychology* **56**, 893–897.

Becker, J. (1974). *Depression: Theory and Research*. Washington, DC: Winston.

Bentler, P.M. (1995). *EQS Structural Equations Program Manual*. Encino, CA: Multivariate Software, Inc.

Binder, D. (1983). On the variances of asymptotically normal estimators from complex surveys. *International Statistical Review* **51**, 279–292.

Birchwood, M., Smith, J., Cochrane, R. *et al.* (1990). The social functioning scale. *British Journal of Psychiatry* **157**, 853–859.

Blalock, H.M. (1964). *Causal Inferences in Nonexperimental Research*. Chapel Hill: University of North Carolina Press.

Blalock, H.M. (1982). *Conceptualization and Measurement in the Social Sciences*. Beverly Hills, CA: Sage.

Bland, J.M. and Altman, D.G. (1986). Statistical methods for assessing agreement between two methods of clinical measurement. *Lancet* **i**, 307–310.

Bollen, K.A. (1984). Multiple indicators: internal consistency or no necessary relationship? *Quality and Quantity* **18**, 377–385.

Bollen, K.A. (1989). *Structural Equation Models with Latent Variables*. New York: Wiley.

Bollen, K.A. and Lennox, R. (1991). Conventional wisdom on measurement: a structural equation perspective. *Psychological Bulletin* **110**, 305–314.

Boyle, G.J. (1985). Self-report measures of depression: some psychometric considerations. *British Journal of Clinical Psychology* **24**, 45–59.

Brett-Jones, J., Garety, P.A. and Hemsley, D. (1987). Measuring delusional experiences: a method and its application. *British Journal of Clinical Psychology* **26**, 257–265.

Brick, J.M. and Kalton, G. (1996). Handling missing data in survey research. *Statistical Methods in Medical Research* **5**, 215–238.

Brown, G.W. and Harris, T. (1978). *Social Origins of Depression*. New York: Free Press.

Brown, W. (1910). Some experimental results in the correlation of mental abilities. *British Journal of Psychology* **3**, 296–322.

Brown, W. (1911). *The Essentials of Mental Measurement*. Cambridge: Cambridge University Press.

Browne, M.W. and Shapiro, A. (1988). Robustness of normal theory methods in the analysis of linear latent variable models. *British Journal of Mathematical and Statistical Psychology* **41**, 193–208.

Buchanan, A., Reed, A., Wesseley, S. *et al.* (1993). Acting on delusions 2: the phenomenological correlates. *British Journal of Psychiatry* **163**, 77–81.

Burt, C. (1940). *The Factors of the Mind*. London: University of London Press.

Burt, C. (1952). Dr William Brown. *British Journal of Psychology, Statistical Section* **5**, 137–138.

Bush, B., Shaw, S., Cleary, P., Delbanco, T.L. and Aronson, M.D. (1987). Screening for alcohol abuse using the CAGE questionnaire. *American Journal of Medicine* **82**, 231–235.

Campbell, D.T. and Fiske, D.W. (1959). Convergent and discriminant validation by the multitrait–multimethod matrix. *Psychological Bulletin* **56**, 81–105.

Carmines, E.G. and Zeller, R.A. (1979). *Reliability and Validity Assessment*. Thousand Oaks, CA: Sage.

Carroll, B.J., Feinberg, M., Gireden, J.F. *et al.* (1982). A specific laboratory test for the diagnosos of melancholia. *Archives of General Psychiatry* **38**, 15–22.

Carroll, R.J., Ruppert, D. and Stefanski, L.A. (1995). *Measurement Error in Non-Linear Models*. London: Chapman & Hall.

Clare, A.W. and Cairns, V.E. (1978). Design, development and the use of a standardized interview to assess social maladjustment and dysfunction in community studies. *Psychological Medicine* **8**, 589–604.

Clayton, D., Spiegelhalter, D., Dunn, G. and Pickles, A. (1998). Analysis of longitudinal binary data from multi-phase sampling (with discussion). *Journal of the Royal Statistical Society B* **60**, 71–102.

Cochran, W.G. (1968). Errors of measurement in statistics. *Technometrics* **10**, 637–666.

Cochran, W.G. (1977). *Sampling Techniques*. New York: Wiley.

Cohen, J. (1960). A coefficient of agreement for nominal scales. *Educational and Psychological Measurement* **20**, 37–46.

Cohen, J. (1968). Weighted kappa: nominal scale agreement with provision for scales disagreement of partial credit. *Psychological Bulletin* **70**, 213–220.

Cole, D.A., Truglio, R. and Peeke, L. (1997). Relation between symptoms of anxiety and depression in children: a multitrait–multimethod–multigroup assessment. *Journal of Consulting and Clinical Psychology* **65**, 110–119.

Cole, D.A., Peeke, L.G., Martin, J.M., Truglio, R. and Seroczynski, A.D. (1998). A longitudinal look at the relation between depression and anxiety in children and adolescents. *Journal of Consulting and Clinical Psychology* **66**, 451–460.

Cox, D.R. and Wermuth, N. (1996). *Multivariate Dependencies*. London: Chapman & Hall.

Cronbach, L.J., Gleser, G.L., Nanda, H. and Rajaratnam, N. (1972). *The Dependability of Behavioral Measurements*. New York: Wiley.

Crow, T.J. (1980). Molecular pathology of schizophrenia: more than a disease process? *British Medical Journal* **280**, 66–68.

Cuzick, J., Edwards, R. and Segnan, N. (1997). Adjusting for non-compliance and contamination in randomized clinical trials. *Statistics in Medicine* **15**, 1017–1029.

Diggle, P. (1998). Dealing with missing values in longitudinal studies. In *Statistical Analysis of Medical Data* (B.S. Everitt and G. Dunn, eds.), pp. 203–228. London: Arnold.

Dohrenwend, B.P. (1995). 'The problem of validity in field studies of Psychological Disorders' revisited. In *Textbook in Psychiatric Epidemiology* (M.T. Tsuang, M. Tohen and G.E.P. Zahner, eds.), pp. 3–20. New York: Wiley-Liss.

Dunn, G. (1989). *Design and Analysis of Reliability Studies*. London: Arnold.

Dunn, G. (1992). Design and analysis of reliability studies. *Statistical Methods in Medical Research* **1**, 123–157.

Dunn, G. (1999). The problem of measurement error in modelling the effect of compliance in a randomized trial. *Statistics in Medicine*, in press.

Dunn, G., Everitt, B. and Pickles, A. (1993). *Modelling Covariances and Latent Variables using EQS*. London: Chapman & Hall.

Dunn, G., Sham, P.C. and Hand, D.J. (1993). Statistics and the nature of depression. *Journal of the Royal Statistical Society, Series A* **156**, 63–87.

Dunn, G., Pickles, A., Tansella, M. and Vázquez-Barquero, J.L. (1999). Two-phase epidemiological surveys in psychiatric research. *British Journal of Psychiatry* **174**, 95–100.

Efron, B. and Feldman, D. (1991). Compliance as an explanatory variable in clinical trials. *Journal of the American Statistical Association* **86**, 9–17.

Ellund, H.B. and Doering, C.R. (1928). The application of statistical method to the study of mental disease. *American Journal of Psychiatry* **84**, 789–808.

Everitt, B.S. (1981). Bimodality and the nature of depression. *British Journal of Psychiatry* **138**, 336–339.

Everitt, B.S. (1987). Statistics in psychiatry. *Statistical Science* **2**, 107–134.

Everitt, B.S. and Dunn, G. (1991). *Applied Multivariate Data Analysis*. London: Arnold.

Everitt, B.S. and Landau, S. (1998). The use of multivariate statistical methods in psychiatry. *Statistical Methods in Medical Research* **7**, 253–277.

Ewing, J.A. (1984). Detecting alcoholism: the CAGE questionnaire. *Journal of the American Medical Association* **252**, 1905–1907.

Eysenck, H.J. (1970). The classification of depressive illness. *British Journal of Psychiatry* **117**, 241–250.

Fayers, P.M. and Hand, D.J. (1997). Factor analysis, causal indicators, and quality of life. *Quality of Life Research* **6**, 139–150.

Fayers, P.M., Hand, D.J., Bjordal, K. and Groenvold, M. (1997). Causal indicators in quality of life research. *Quality of Life Research* **6**, 393–406.

Fisher, R.A. (1942). *The Design of Experiments* (3rd edition). Edinburgh: Oliver & Boyd.

Fitzmaurice, G.M., Laird, N.M., Zahner, G.E.P. and Daskalis, C. (1995). Bivariate logistic regression analysis of childhood psychopathology ratings using multiple informants. *American Journal of Epidemiology* **142**, 1194–1203.

Fleiss, J.L. (1972). Classification of depressive disorders by numerical typology. *Journal of Psychiatric Research* **9**, 141–153.

Fleiss, J.L. (1981). Balanced incomplete blocks designs for inter-rater reliability studies. *Applied Psychological Measurement* **5**, 105–112.

Fleiss, J.L. (1987). *The Design and Analysis of Clinical Experiments*. New York: Wiley.

Fleiss, J.L. and Cuzick, J. (1979). The reliability of dichotomous judgements: unequal numbers of judgements per subject. *Applied Psychological Measurement* **3**, 537–542.

Fuller, W.A. (1987). *Measurement Error Models*. New York: Wiley.

Goldberg, D.P. (1972). *The Detection of Psychiatric Illness by Questionnaire*. London: Oxford University Press.

Goldberg, D.P. and Williams, P. (1988). *The User's Guide to the General Health Questionnaire*. London: NFER/Nelson.

Goldberg, D.P., Cooper, B., Eastwood, M.R., Kedwood, H.B. and Shepherd, M. (1970). A standardised psychiatric interview for use in community surveys. *British Journal of Preventative and Social Medicine* **24**, 18–23.

Gornbein, J.A., Lazarro, C.G. and Little, R.J.A. (1992). Incomplete data in repeated measures analysis. *Statistical Methods in Medical Research* **1**, 275–295.

Grayson, D.A. (1987). Can categorical and dimensional views of psychiatric illness be distinguished? *British Journal of Psychiatry* **151**, 355–361.

Hamilton, M. (1960). A rating scale for depression. *Journal of Neurology Neurosurgery and Psychiatry* **23**, 56–61.

Hamilton, M. (1967). Development of a rating scale for primary depressive illness. *British Journal of Social and Clinical Psychology* **6**, 278–296.

Hanley, J.A. and McNeill, B.J. (1982). The meaning and use of the area under a receiver operating characteristic curve. *Radiology* **143**, 29–36.

Hart, B. and Spearman, C. (1912). General ability, its existence and nature. *British Journal of Psychology* **9**, 51–84.

Healy, M.J.R. (1969). Contribution to the discussion, in Moran (1969), pp. 517–520.

Heise, D.R. (1969). Separating reliability and stability in test–retest correlation. *American Sociological Review* **34**, 93–101.

Hewitt, J.K., Silberg, J.L., Neale, M.C., Eaves, L.J. and Erickson, M. (1992). The analysis of parental ratings of children's behavior using LISREL. *Behavior Genetics* **22**, 293–317.

Huber, P. (1967). The behavior of maximum likelihood estimates under nonstandard conditions. In *Proceedings of the 5th Berkeley Symposium on Mathematical Statistics and Probability*, Vol. 1, pp. 221–233. Berkeley: University of California Press.

Hustig, H.H. and Hafner, R.J. (1990). Persistent auditory hallucinations and their relationship to delusions and mood. *Journal of Nervous and Mental Disease* **178**, 264–267.

Jasper, H.H. (1930). The measurement of depression–elation and its relation to a measure of extraversion–introversion. *Journal of Abnormal Social Psychology* **25**, 307–318.

Johnson, T. (1998). Clinical trials in psychiatry: background and statistical perspective. *Statistical Methods in Medical Research* **7**, 209–234.

Kelley, T.L. (1923). *Statistical Method*. New York: Macmillan.

Kendell, R.E. (1968). *The Classification of Depressive Illness*. Oxford: Oxford University Press.

Kendell, R.E. (1976). The classification of depression: a review of contemporary confusion. *British Journal of Psychiatry* **129**, 15–28.

Kendler, K.S., Neale, M., Kessler, R., Heath, A. and Eaves, L. (1993). A twin study of recent life events and difficulties. *Archives of General Psychiatry* **50**, 789–796.

Kenny, D.A. and Kashy, D.A. (1992). Analysis of multitrait–multimethod matrix by confirmatory factor analysis. *Psychological Bulletin* **112**, 165–172.

Kessler, R.C. (1994). The National Comorbidity Survey of the United States. *International Review of Psychiatry* **6**, 365–376.

Kovacs, M. (1981). Rating scales to assess depression in school-aged children. *Acta Paedopsychiatrica* **46**, 305–315.

Kraemer, H.C. (1992). *Statistical Evaluation of Medical Tests*. Thousand Oaks, CA: Sage.

Kraemer, H.C., Pruyn, J.P., Gibbons, R.D., Greenhouse, J.B., Grochocinski, V.J., Waternaux, C. and Kupfer, D.J. (1987). Methodology in psychiatric research: report on the 1986 MacArthur Foundation network I methodology Institute. *Archives of General Psychiatry* **44**, 1100–1106.

Kramer, M. (1989). The biostatistical approach. In *The Scope of Epidemiological Psychiatry* (P. Williams, G. Wilkinson and K. Rawnsley, eds.), pp. 86–107. London: Routledge.

Kuipers, E., Garety, P., Fowler, D., Dunn, G., Bebbington, P., Freeman, D. and Hadley, C. (1997). London–East Anglia randomised controlled trial of cognitive-behavioural therapy for psychosis. I: effects of the treatment phase. *British Journal of Psychiatry* **171**, 319–327.

Lavange, L.M., Keyes, L.L., Koch, G.G. and Margolis, P.A. (1994). Application of sample survey methods for modeling ratios to incidence densities. *Statistics in Medicine* **13**, 342–355.

Lehtonen, R. and Pahkinen, E.J. (1995). *Practical Methods for Design and Analysis of Complex Surveys*. Chichester: Wiley.

Lewis, A.J. (1946). On the place of physical treatment in psychiatry. *British Medical Bulletin* **3**, 22–24.

Lewis, G., Pelosi, A.J., Araya, R. and Dunn, G. (1992). Measuring psychiatric disorder in the community: a standardised assessment for use by lay interviewers. *Psychological Medicine* **22**, 465–486.

Liang, K.Y. and Zeger, S.L. (1986). Longitudinal data analysis using generalized linear models. *Biometrika* **73**, 13–22.

Little, R.J.A. and Rubin, D.B. (1987). *Statistical Analysis with Missing Data*. New York: Wiley.

Lord, F.M. and Novick, M.R. (1968). *Statistical Theories of Mental Test Scores*. Reading, MA: Addison-Wesley.

MacCallum, R.C. and Browne, M.W. (1993). The use of causal indicators in covariance structure models: some practical issues. *Psychological Bulletin* **114**, 533–541.

Mapother, E. (1928). Review of *The Abilities of Man* by C. Spearman. *Journal of Mental Science* **74**, 113–119.

Maxwell, A.E. (1972). Difficulties in the dimensional description of symptomatology. *British Journal of Psychiatry* **121**, 19–26.

Mayer, J.M. (1978). Assessment of depression. In *Advances in Psychological Assessment* (P. McReynolds, ed.), Vol. 4, pp. 368–425. Washington, DC: Jossey-Bass.

Messer, S.C. and Gross, A.M. (1994). Childhood depression and aggression: a covariance structure analysis. *Behavior Research and Therapy* **32**, 633–677.

Milbank Memorial Fund Commission (1972). *Higher Education in Public Health*. New York: Prodist.

Moran, P.A.P. (1969). Statistical methods in psychiatric research (with discussion). *Journal of the Royal Statistical Society A* **132**, 484–525.

Mowbray, R.M. (1972). The Hamilton Rating Scale for depression: a factor analysis. *Psychological Medicine* **2**, 272–280.

Murphy, E.A. (1964). One cause?, many causes?: the argument from the bimodal distribution. *Journal of Chronic Disease* **17**, 301–324.

Murphy, J.M. (1995). Diagnostic interviews and rating scales in adult psychiatry. In *Textbook in Psychiatric Epidemiology* (M.T. Tsuang, M. Tohen and G.E.P. Zahner, eds.), pp. 253–271. New York: Wiley-Liss.

Overall, J.E. and Gorham, D.R. (1962). The Brief Psychiatric Rating Scale. *Psychological Reports* **10**, 799–812.

Paykel, E.S. (1981). Have multivariate statistics contributed to classification? *British Journal of Psychiatry* **139**, 357–362.

Pepe, M.S., Reilly, M. and Fleming, T.R. (1994). Auxiliary outcome data and the mean score method. *Journal of Statistical Planning and Inference* **42**, 137–160.

Piccinelli, M., Pini, S., Bonizzato, P., Paltrinieri, E., Saltini, A., Scantamburlo, L., Bellantuono, C. and Tansella, M. (1995). Results from the Verona Centre. In *Mental Illness in General Health Care: An International Study* (T.B. Üstön and N. Sartorius, eds.). New York: Wiley.

Pickering, G.W. (1968). *High Blood Pressure*. Edinburgh: Churchill Livingstone.

Pickles, A. (1998). Clinical epidemiology. *Statistical Methods in Medical Research* **7**, 235–251.

Pickles, A. and Dunn, G. (1998). Estimation of disease prevalence from screening data. In *Encylopedia of Biostatistics* (P. Armitage and T. Colton, eds.), Vol. 5, pp. 3484–3490. Chichester: Wiley.

Pickles, A., Dunn, G. and Vázquez-Barquero, J.L. (1995). Screening for stratification in two-phase ('two-stage') epidemiological surveys. *Statistical Methods in Medical Research* **4**, 73–89.

Plomin, R. (1994). *Genetics and Experience: The Interplay between Nature and Nurture*. Thousand Oaks, CA: Sage.

Plomin, R., Litchenstein, P., Pedersen, N.L., McClearn, G.E. and Nesselroade, J.R. (1990). Genetic influences on life events during the last half of the life span. *Psychology and Aging* **5**, 25–30.

Radloff, L.S. (1977). The CES-D Scale: a self-report depression scale for research in the general population. *Applied Psychological Measurement* **1**, 385–401.

Rasch, G. (1960). *Probabilistic Models for Some Intelligence and Attainment Tests*. Copenhagen: Danish Institute for Educational Research.

Reilly, M. and Pepe, M. (1997). The relationship between hot-deck multiple imputation and weighted likelihood. *Statistics in Medicine* **16**, 5–19.

Reynolds, C.R. and Richmond, B.O. (1978). What I think and feel: a revised measure of children's manifest anxiety. *Journal of Abnormal Child Psychology* **6**, 271–280.

Rindskopf, D. (1992). A general approach to categorical data analysis with missing data, using generalized linear models with composite links. *Psychometrika* **57**, 29–42.

Robins, L.N., Helzer, J., Croughan, J. and Ratcliff, K.S. (1981). The NIMH Diagnostic Interview Schedule: its history, characteristics and validity. *Archives of General Psychiatry* **38**, 381–389.

Robins, L.N., Wing, J.K., Wittchen, H.U., Helzer, J.E., Babor, T.F., Burke, J., Farmer, A., Jablenski, A., Pickens, R., Regier, D.A., Sartorius, N. and Towle, L.H. (1988). The Composite International Diagnostic Interview Schedule: an epidemiologic instrument suitable for use in conjunction with different diagnostic systems and in different cultures. *Archives of General Psychiatry* **45**, 1069–1077.

Rose, G. (1989). The mental health of populations. In *The Scope of Epidemiological Psychiatry* (P. Williams, G. Wilkinson and K. Rawnsley, eds.), pp. 77–85. London: Routledge.

Rose, G. (1992). *The Strategy of Preventative Medicine*. Oxford: Oxford University Press.

Rumke, H.C. (1960). *Psychiatrie*, Vol. 2, Amsterdam: Scheltema & Holkema.

Särndal, C.-E., Swensson, B. and Wretman, J. (1992). *Model Assisted Survey Sampling*. New York: Springer.

Satorra, A. and Bentler, P.M. (1990). Model conditions for asymptotic robustness in the analysis of linear relations. *Computational Statistics and Data Analysis* **10**, 235–249.

Scott, W.A. (1955). Reliability of content analysis: the case of nominal scale coding. *Public Opinion Quarterly* **19**, 321–325.

Schouten, H.J.A. (1985). Statistical measurement of interobserver agreement. Unpublished doctoral dissertation. Rotterdam: Erasmus University.

Shah, B.V., Folsom, R.E., Lavange, L.M., Wheeless, S.C., Boyle, K.E. and Williams, R.L. (1993). *Statistical Methods and Mathematical Algorithms used in SUDAAN*. Research Triangle Park, North Carolina: Research Triangle Institute.

Sham, P. (1998). *Statistics in Human Genetics*. London: Arnold.

Shavelson, R.J. and Webb, N.M. (1991). *Generalizability Theory: A Primer*. Newbury Park, CA: Sage.

Shrout, P.E. (1998). Measurement reliability and agreement in psychiatry. *Statistical Methods in Medical Research* **7**, 301–317.

Shrout, P.E. and Fleiss, J.L. (1981). Intra-class correlations: uses in assessing rater reliability. *Psychological Bulletin* **86**, 420–428.

Simins, C. (1933). Studies in experimental psychiatry: IV. Deterioration of 'G' in psychotic patients. *Journal of Mental Science* **79**, 704–734.

Simonoff, E., Pickles, A., Hewitt, J., Silberg, J., Rutter, M., Loeber, R., Meyer, J., Neale, M. and Eaves, L. (1995). Multiple raters of disruptive child behavior: using a genetic strategy to examine shared views and bias. *Behavior Genetics* **25**, 311–326.

Somer, A. and Zeger, S.L. (1991). On estimating efficacy from clinical trials. *Statistics in Medicine* **10**, 45–52.

Spearman, C. (1904). General intelligence objectively determined and measured. *American Journal of Psychology* **15**, 201–293.

Spearman, C. (1910). Correlation calculated from faulty date. *British Journal of Psychology* **3**, 271–295.

Spearman, C. (1927). *The Abilities of Man*. New York: Macmillan.

Spearman, C. (1929). The tenth Maudsley Lecture: the psychiatric use of the methods and results of experimental psychology. *Journal of Mental Science* **75**, 357–370.

StataCorp (1997) *Stata Statistical Software: Release 5.0*. College Station, TX: Stata Corporation.

Stephenson, W. (1931). Studies in experimental psychiatry: I. A case of general inertia. *Journal of Mental Science* **77**, 723–741.

Stephenson, W. (1932a). Studies in experimental psychiatry: II. Some contact of *p*-factor with psychiatry. *Journal of Mental Science* **78**, 315–330.

Stephenson, W. (1932b). Studies in experimental psychiatry: III. *p*-Score and inhibition for high-*p* praecox cases. *Journal of Mental Science* **78**, 908–928.

Streiner, D.L. and Norman, G.R. (1995). *Health Measurement Scales: a Practical Guide to their Development and Use* (2nd edition). Oxford: Oxford University Press.

Studman, I.G. (1935). Studies in experimental psychiatry. V. 'W' and 'F' factors in relation to traits of personality. *Journal of Mental Science* **81**, 107–137.

Tarnopolsky, A., Hand, D.J., McLean, E.K., Roberts, H. and Wiggins, R.D. (1979). Validity and uses of a screening questionnaire (GHQ) in the community. *British Journal of Psychiatry* **134**, 508–515.

Thapar, A. and McGuffin, P. (1996). Genetic influences on life events in childhood. *Psychological Medicine* **26**, 813–820.

Thompson, R. and Baker, R.J. (1981). Composite link functions in generalized linear models. *Applied Statistics* **30**, 125–131.

Thornicroft, G. and Tansella, M. (eds.) (1996). *Mental Health Outcome Measures.* Berlin: Springer.

Urquhart, J. and De Klerk, E. (1998). Contending paradigms for the interpretation of data on patient compliance with therapeutic drug regimens. *Statistics in Medicine* **17**, 251–267.

Van der Does, A.J.W., Dingemanns, P.M.A.J., Linszen, D.H., Nugter, M.A. and Scholte, W.F. (1995). Dimensions and subtypes of recent-onset schizophrenia. A longitudinal analysis. *Journal of Nervous and Mental Disease* **183**, 681–687.

Vázquez-Barquero, J.L., Diez-Manrique, J.F., Pena, C., Quintanal, R.G. and Labrador Lopez, M. (1986). Two stage design in a community survey. *British Journal of Psychiatry* **149**, 88–97.

Vázquez-Barquero, J.L., Lastra, I., Cuesta Nuñez, M.J., Herrerra Castanedo, S. and Dunn, G. (1996). Patterns of positive and negative symptoms in first episode schizophrenia. *British Journal of Psychiatry* **168**, 693–701.

Vázquez-Barquero, J.L., Garcia, J., Artal Simón, J., Iglesias, C., Montejo, J., Herrán, A. and Dunn, G. (1997). Mental health in primary care. An epidemiological study of morbidity and use of health resources. *British Journal of Psychiatry* **170**, 529–535.

Von Korff, M. and Üstün, T.B. (1995). Methods of the WHO Collaborative Study on 'Psychological Problems in General Health Care'. In *Mental Illness in General Health Care: An International Study* (T.B. Üstün and N. Sartorius, eds.), pp. 19–38. New York: Wiley.

Weckowicz, T.E., Muir, W. and Cropley, A. (1978). A factor analysis of the Beck inventory of depression. *Journal of Consulting Psychology* **87**, 155–164.

Wheaton, B. (1985). Models for the stress-buffering functions of coping resources. *Journal of Health and Social Behavior* **26**, 352–364.

White, H. (1982). Maximum likelihood estimation for mis-specified models. *Econometrics* **50**, 1–25.

Wiley, D.E. and Wiley, J.A. (1970). The estimation of measurement error in panel data. *American Sociological Review* **35**, 112–117.

Wing, J.K. (1983). The use and misuse of the PSE. *British Journal of Psychiatry* **143**, 111–117.

Wing, J.K. (1994). Relevance of psychiatric epidemiology to clinical psychiatry. *International Reviews of Psychiatry* **6**, 259–264.

Wing, J. (1996). SCAN (Schedules for Clinical Assessment in Neuropsychiatry) and the PSE (Present State Examination) tradition. In Thornicroft and Tansella (eds.) (1996), pp. 123–130.

Wing, J.K., Cooper, J.E. and Sartorius, N. (1974). *The Description and Classification of Psychiatric Symptoms. An Instructional Manual for the PSE and CATEGO System.* Cambridge: Cambridge University Press.

Wing, J.K., Babor, T., Brugha, T., Burke, J., Cooper, J., Giel, R., Jablensky, A., Regier, D. and Sartorius, N. (1990). SCAN schedules for clinical assessment in neuropsychiatry. *Archives of General Psychiatry* **47**, 589–593.

World Health Organisation (1992). *SCAN Schedules for Clinical Assessment in Neuropsychiatry.* Geneva: WHO.

Wynn-Jones, L.L. (1928). An investigation into the significance of perseveration. *Journal of Mental Science* **74**, 653–659.

Yule, G.U. (1911). *An Introduction to the Theory of Statistics.* London: Griffin.

Zeger, S.L. and Liang, K.Y. (1991). Dose–response estimands. *Journal of the American Statistical Association* **86**, 18–19.

Zelen, M. (1979). A new design for randomized clinical trials. *New England Journal of Medicine* **300**, 1242–1245.

Zhou, X.H. (1996). Nonparametric ML estimate of an ROC area corrected for verification bias. *Biometrics* **52**, 310–316.

Zhou, X.H. (1998). Correcting for verification bias in studies of a diagnostic test's accuracy. *Statistical Methods in Medical Research* **7**, 337–353.

Zigmond, A.S. and Snaith, R.P. (1983). The Hospital Anxiety and Depression Scale. *Acta Psychiatrica Scandinavica* **67**, 361–370.

Index